D1486128

THE CLUMSY CHILD

Volume 5 in the Series

Major Problems in Neurology

JOHN N. WALTON, TD, MD, DSc, FRCP
Consulting Editor

OTHER MONOGRAPHS IN THE SERIES

PUBLISHED

Barnett, Foster and Hudgson: **Syringomyelia,** *1973*
Dubowitz and Brooke: **Muscle Biopsy: A Modern Approach,** *1973*
Pallis and Lewis: **The Neurology of Gastrointestinal Disease,** *1974*
Hutchinson and Acheson: **Strokes,** *1975*

FORTHCOMING

Behan and Currie: **Neuroimmunology**
Cartlidge and Shaw: **Medical Aspects of Head Injury**
Newson Davis and Cameron: **The Neurology of Breathing and its Disorders**

The Clumsy Child

*A Study of Developmental Apraxic
and Agnosic Ataxia*

SASSON S. GUBBAY, MD(W.A.), BS (Adel.), FRACP

*Neurologist, Princess Margaret Hospital for Children and
Perth Medical Centre; Assistant Neurologist, Royal Perth
Hospital; Clinical Lecturer in Neurology, Department of
Medicine, University of Western Australia; Honorary Schools
Medical Officer.*

1975

W. B. Saunders Company Ltd   London · Philadelphia · Toronto

W. B. Saunders Company Ltd: 1 St Anne's Road
Eastbourne, East Sussex BN21 3UN

West Washington Square
Philadelphia, PA 19105

833 Oxford Street
Toronto, Ontario M8Z 5T9

Library of Congress Cataloging in Publication Data

Gubbay, Sasson S.
The clumsy child.
Bibliography: p. 177
Includes index.
1. Child development deviations. 2. Apraxia.
3. Ataxia. 4. Agnosia. I. Title. [DNLM:
1. Apraxia—In infancy and childhood. 2. Movement
disorders—In infancy and childhood. WL340 G921c]
RJ135.G82   618.9'28'5884   75–12487
ISBN 0-7216-4340-X

Printed by The Whitefriars Press Ltd, London and Tonbridge

Print Number: 9 8 7 6 5 4 3 2

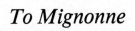

To Mignonne

Foreword

The term 'minimal cerebral dysfunction' was introduced some years ago to identify a group of children showing a variety of executive and cognitive defects, often in the absence of conclusive evidence indicative of perinatal brain damage or cerebral palsy. Many authors have subsequently argued cogently that the term is unsatisfactory as a diagnostic label and that in such children it is better to identify the specific defects which are present in each individual case and to include these under the generic title of 'specific learning disabilities'. Whereas various developmental disorders of speech, as well as reading disability (developmental dyslexia) have been recognised for many years, less attention has been paid until comparatively recently to the various defects of execution and cognition which may occur in otherwise apparently normal children and which may lead to abnormalities of motor development and performance. In general these are often 'clumsy children' and in this stimulating monograph Dr Gubbay analyses the nature, causation and management of this syndrome lucidly, succinctly and yet comprehensively.

He begins with a discussion of the many neurological disorders which may cause abnormalities of motor development, before going on to delineate the specific clinical features of that abnormal degree of clumsiness with retarded physical development in otherwise intelligent children which has been called 'developmental apraxia and agnosia' or 'developmental apraxic ataxia'. He then reviews some early investigations which he carried out upon a group of such children in Newcastle upon Tyne, and goes on to describe the methods and results of a comprehensive survey which he subsequently performed in a large number of schoolchildren in Western Australia. This latter investigation confirmed his view that various degrees of the syndrome are common in the apparently normal school population and may give rise to substantial difficulties in learning and associated behavioural abnormalities. He describes in detail a number of simple clinical tests which he has devised in order to identify children suffering from this type of abnormality and goes on to give a great deal of useful information about methods of assessment and management of such patients. This clearly written monograph, based upon a great deal of quantitative information which has been carefully analysed, highlights a clinical syndrome which has often been neglected in the past by paediatricians, neurologists, psychiatrists and schoolteachers alike. To all of these groups, Dr Gubbay's thorough consideration of the problem, supported by a careful analysis of the relevant literature and enlivened by the fruits of his own experience, will be of great interest. Acceptance of his wise counsel will undoubtedly do a great deal to identify these children who, through no fault of their own, have often appeared to be misfits in our modern society, and will also do much to help them to overcome the disabilities which are so mysterious to the casual examiner and yet so easy to understand and sometimes to alleviate when appreciated by the initiated.

Newcastle upon Tyne, 1975   John N. Walton

Preface

Many varied disorders of the nervous system interfere with motor performance in children. Of special interest is the child with clumsiness arising from a failure of the development of normal praxis. Such clumsiness is often observed within the symptomatology of 'minimal cerebral dysfunction'. (The word 'ataxia' in the sub-title of this book is discussed under 'Definitions' in Chapter 2 and is purely descriptive, referring to the unsteady or inco-ordinate movements of these youngsters.) We are all familiar with the wide variations in dexterity and gracefulness in individual children. In some cases of relative indexterity there is a readily recognisable neurological basis either because of a history of neurological disease or the presence of demonstrable conventional neurological signs. Other children fail to develop normal physical skills because of an intrinsic impairment of central nervous system organisation. Because of the lack of obvious neurological evidence, these children frequently are not recognised as suffering from a congenital encephalopathy. Undue stresses may result when they are therefore unjustly expected to conform to normal achievement standards, often with subsequent educational and behavioural aberration.

One might well ask why developmental clumsiness should be treated as a separate entity within the field of minimal cerebral dysfunction or specific learning disability. The answer is simply that there should be a concerted effort to sift out the very complex issues applying to neuro-developmental disorders. With the advent of extremely successful preventative medical programmes in Western countries, the orientation of the paediatrician in the last few decades has gradually moved towards community welfare and broader issues of child care. Consequently when learning and developmental problems in children were brought into focus it was appreciated that at least five per cent of the juvenile population were involved in some way. Because very large numbers of children must be considered, it has become necessary to resort to reclassification in order to study specific problems in greater depth. Surely the time has come for us to heed the advice of Walzer and Richmond (1973) who consider that we clearly need a taxonomy for this group of disorders.

A survey of one thousand schoolchildren is described and reveals that a significant number of apparently normal children attending ordinary schools have problems related to inefficient motor function. The clumsiness exhibited by the large majority of these children was due to a failure of the development of praxis, which can be designated 'developmental apraxic ataxia'. A simple standardised battery of eight tests has been developed to facilitate recognition of such children. It is suggested that these standardised tests of motor aptitude should be used by medical practitioners including paediatricians, paediatric neurologists and school medical officers as an adjunct to routine neurological examination. Some observations, potentially of considerable philosophical interest, are made on the pathogenesis of developmental apraxia. The management of these children, a much greater challenge, is discussed in detail.

The author hopes that the orientation of the book has been towards the needs of medical practitioners and that it might serve as a reference for the educationist, psychologist and therapist.

I am most grateful for the introduction to *The Clumsy Child* by my former chief, Professor John N. Walton, and for his encouragement in the preparation of this work. Much of the material in Chapter 3 has been published previously in *Brain* with my co-authors, Professors Walton and Court and Dr Ellis, who were instrumental in delineating the entity of 'Developmental Apraxia and Agnosia'. Some of the work reported is based upon my thesis for the Degree of Doctor of Medicine submitted to the University of Western Australia. Due acknowledgement is made to the Editor and publishers of *Brain* and also to the Editor and publishers of the *Proceedings of the Australian Association of Neurologists, Neurology* (India) and the *Medical Journal of Australia* for material given in Chapters 3 and 4.

I am also indebted to Associate Professor N. Stenhouse for his general advice regarding the design of the survey and for the assistance of his Department in the statistical analyses. Mr R. B. van Raalte of the Department of Medical Illustration at Royal Perth Hospital assisted materially with excellent illustrations and photography. Immense assistance from official channels was obtained through the very kind efforts of the previous Director of School Medical Services, Dr A. R. Edmonds, who initiated my appointment as Honorary Schools Medical Officer which facilitated my access to the schoolchildren. It was most encouraging to receive every support at the outset from Dr D. Mossenson, Assistant Director General of Education and Mr S. Wallace, previous Director of Primary School Education; and from Messrs L. G. Baker and K. Gosling of the Guidance and Special Education Branch of the Education Department for the intelligence tests. I am particularly grateful for the advice and assistance from all the principals of the five schools which were involved in the study and to the schoolteachers who gave their time to complete the questionnaires. This work would not have been possible without the friendly co-operation of the pupils and their parents.

Professors R. A. Joske, A. J. Yates, W. B. Macdonald and Associate Professor M. G. McCall gave helpful advice and encouragement during the planning phase of the research project. Dr B. Lanzrein assisted with the translations of the European literature, and Miss M. A. Gillett of the Medical Library of Western Australia rendered valuable assistance with the bibliography.

My secretaries, Mrs Sandra Goodwin and Mrs Shirley Smith, through their efficiency have made my task very much easier and Mrs Goodwin also assisted with some of the screening examinations. The electroencephalograms were performed by Miss Helen Macintyre and Mrs Lynn Nunn at Princess Margaret Hospital for Children, and by Miss B. P. Longley at the Regional Neurological Centre at Newcastle upon Tyne; and I am indebted to the administration of these hospitals for allowing me the use of their facilities. Dr David D. Barwick assisted with the interpretation of the 21 Newcastle electroencephalograms. I must record my gratitude to Professor H. Waring who encouraged me greatly and gave me tremendous moral support.

This study was in part supported by grants obtained from the Princess Margaret Children's Medical Research Foundation and the Royal Australasian College of Physicians.

Perth, Western Australia, 1975   Sasson S. Gubbay

Contents

CHAPTER ONE

Clumsiness in Childhood

We are all familiar with the wide variation in the degree of dexterity and gracefulness of normal children. Acts of juvenile agility such as the poise of the little ballet dancer or the nimbleness of the gymnast are sometimes beheld with wonderment. The parent who is favoured with a child exhibiting superior abilities at sport, music or constructional hobbies soon recognises that much of the gift is an intrinsic quality. In some instances high aspirations and diligence in the child are rewarded with success. In many other cases, despite dogged determination and enthusiastic practice, nothing more than mediocrity is achieved.

The clumsy antics of the toddler or the younger child may well be a source of genuine mirth and may even be acclaimed by a doting parent as an appealing characteristic. Few teachers and fewer parents show much anxiety over kindergarten children with non-progressive clumsiness. Such is a perfectly healthy attitude because with maturation the large majority of less dexterous children achieve acceptable levels of motor functioning without any conscious effort at improvement. Even in older children attending primary and perhaps early secondary school, a minor degree of ineptness at sport, gymnastics or dancing may be perfectly acceptable. The bespectacled, myopic, studious youth may eventually become diffident in taking up his sporting activities, especially if he can compensate adequately for this deficiency by his more intellectual pursuits. Indeed a poor performance in certain physical activities may be assumed as an affectation. Boys often have no wish to excel at dancing and may even consider their masculinity to be at stake if they show themselves to be nimble on their feet. Yet there is always the child who anticipates his inferior performance at physical activities with anguish for he knows that he is readily ridiculed by his fellows or perhaps by his teacher.

What do we mean by *clumsiness* in a child? No creature could be clumsier than the newborn baby. We can hardly designate the groping movements of the infant or the failure of a five-year-old child to tie shoelaces as clumsy acts. Small children cannot hope to emulate the mundane physical skills embodied in the everyday activities of their older siblings. Surely clumsiness, like intelligence, is a comparative term contingent upon normally accepted standards which increase with chronological age. The term 'clumsy child' could be expressed more aptly as 'abnormally clumsy child', for clumsiness is an accepted feature of childhood just as mutism is of infancy.

Abnormal clumsiness in children occurs for a large variety of reasons, but when the clumsiness is isolated and apparently constitutional,there is still much speculation as to pathophysiology. Some authors select clumsiness as the central feature of a syndrome and hence the designation 'clumsy children'. Others regard clumsiness as a manifestation of a broader concept of dysfunction affecting all skills that have developed as part of the total intellect and hence the term 'minimal cerebral dysfunction'. Thus a child with a widespread physiological defect of cerebral organisation might manifest mental retardation which includes an associated clumsiness, whereas another child with simply a developmental right–left disorientation or alternatively an isolated apraxic disorder might manifest a similar degree of clumsiness for quite different reasons. Yet another child with a structural organic disturbance of the brain, which may be progressive or non-progressive, may exhibit signs of a classical neurological disturbance resulting in defective motor performance. Clumsiness could be regarded therefore as an all-inclusive end-product of differing aetiologies implying heterogenous pathophysiology.

The integrity of many differing neurological functions are necessary for the execution of skilled movements. The intactness of pyramidal, extrapyramidal and sensory pathways are not even as fundamental as the basic factors of consciousness, intelligence and the ability to plan motor activity. The essence of awareness and experience is consciousness. Any reduction of the conscious level, as in physiological drowsiness or pathological states, as exemplified by various metabolic disorders, results in unsteadiness akin to drunkenness. Subtle degrees of loss of alertness may not be fully appreciated especially in test situations. The child on anticonvulsant, sedative or tranquilliser medication is always viewed with caution by the experienced professional who deals with children. If consciousness is dependent upon the alerting effect of the reticular formation upon the cerebral cortical functions, then the integrity of the cerebral cortical neurones themselves is obviously also of profound importance. Whereas a depression of reticular activation may result in a depression of consciousness, a primary diffuse reduction of cortical activity results in inferior intellectual performance. As motor planning itself is an intellectual function, the child with congenital or acquired intellectual retardation will usually be clumsy even when neurological physical examination reveals no evidence of cranial nerve, motor or sensory dysfunction.

The mentally deficient child will exhibit increasing degrees of awkwardness for increasing complexities of intellectually challenging physical tasks. This lack of praxis is no more specific for such a child than might be a similar lack of phasis or gnosis, and it therefore must not be designated as apraxia any more than its defective speech or visuo-spatial functions might be alluded to as aphasia or agnosia. Where a series of movements requires no real challenge to motor planning for a child with intellectual retardation there is no real clumsiness. Automatic movements such as walking or running may be executed perfectly. The breakdown of well-integrated movement, however simple, occurs when it has to be learned rather than repeated from former experience.

Praxis sometimes has been defined as the ability to 'motor plan'. It implies, firstly, that there must be a motivation to plan, and secondly, that the subject is able to produce skilled movement through the facilitation of synaptic transmission along stereotyped pathways at all levels within the central nervous system. These levels include cortex, basal ganglia, cerebellum and brainstem acting upon final common pathways through the spinal cord and peripheral nerves. The facilitation of specific pathways comes about through kinaesthetic feedback from the periphery largely through the medium of 'haptic' processing, or the integration of sensory input into the central nervous system. It is likely that these feedback mechanisms result in positive effects from inhibitory neurones and synapses as well as positive effects from facilitatory synapses. How this input is translated into the semi-permanent changes that occur at neuronal level is very much a matter of contention, but forms the basis of the memory system of the brain. There must be a chemical change occurring in the neuronal nucleus which ultimately alters the physical property of any one cell in a particular synaptic chain.

The integrity of neuronal function and circuitry is not an 'all-or-nothing' affair. Relative impairment may be an intrinsic property in one particular individual and not the result of destructive processes as occur in encephaloclastic disease. Comparatively large areas of brain may be destroyed through disease processes in the fetus or young child, but the transference of their function to other areas of the cortex in particular may result in the apparent restoration of neurological competence. However, it is idle to pretend that even small areas of damage to the cerebral cortical substance can be fully compensated by this transference of function, because in the final analysis the total number of neurones is less and the cerebral reserve at least is reduced. In most cases it is not possible to predict what might have been the normal function of such a brain, for its performance may still be within the limits of normality.

The smooth functioning of the motor system not only depends upon its anatomical intactness, but also upon the integrity of all other central structures which act upon or influence motor function. Thus virtually any disturbance of the nervous system, most particularly disorders of the motor system, will result in abnormal clumsiness. To appreciate fully the impact of a physiologically incompetent motor system which results in indexterity of pathological proportions, we must consider the effect of all pathological influences upon motor functioning.

The pragmatic approach of the neurologist has been inculcated largely by his critical observations of clinicopathological relationships. The separation of clinical neurology from psychiatry has been influenced by anatomical and later by biochemical and electrophysiological analyses of disturbed function. Until relatively recently the neurologist has not been so concerned with how the brain actually works except in broad philosophical overtones. He has accepted the normal functioning as a fact—even as axiomatic—and has been preoccupied rather with its abnormal function as the result of demonstrable pathological processes. Thus schizophrenic disease will remain within the province of the psychiatrist at least as long as an organic pathological basis remains elusive. Demonstrable organic changes which produce clumsiness in the broader sense of the term, such as may occur with spasticity, hemiparesis, ataxia and abnormal movement, are responsible for their unmistakable inclusion within neurological territory. Where no definite pathological disturbances have been found, as with developmental neurological dysfunctions including develop- mental dyslexia and developmental apraxia, a neurological basis has also been accepted. However, these are examples of conditions which are neurologically imprecise rather than distinct neurological entities and hence may be relegated to the borderlands of neurology until they can be defined by pathologically acceptable parameters.

It is appropriate now to consider comprehensively all the causes of clumsiness in children. Abnormal clumsiness may arise from virtually any disturbance of the nervous system, and not exclusively when there is disruption of the motor system.

MOTOR DEFECTS IN CHILDREN

Classically the motor system is considered as comprising pyramidal and ex- trapyramidal components. However, disorders of motor function have a more widespread pathophysiological basis than malfunction of either the pyramidal or extrapyramidal pathways, for these systems may be even profoundly modified by visual, sensory and labyrinthine dysfunction. When thinking in terms of clinical neurological function it is often inappropriate to consider any part of the nervous system in isolation, for the central nervous system might be regarded as a nerve network where activation in any one area has widespread implications regarding factors of input, output, facilitation and inhibition. The integrity of the nerve network is partly dependent upon inbuilt heredoevolutionary factors and partly upon the acquisition of newer functions facilitated by environmental experiences. The fundamental difference between developmental and acquired neurological dysfunction is that the latter implies the loss of previously intact functions from a pathological process. In developmental dysfunction, the particular function under consideration has never developed normally, either because of an impairment of innate cerebral mechanisms or the understimulation of an otherwise intact network owing to faulty input pathways. There may even be deprivation of the individual from normal environmental influences usually obtained through parents and teachers. Acquired neurological dysfunction tends to be more circumscribed in its clinical effects, just as it is more circumscribed in a pathological sense than developmental dysfunction where presumably there is a more diffuse disruption of the nerve network.

In general, motor defects in children can be considered in either (1) progressive or (2) non-progressive categories. At the time of original presentation rapidly progressive disorders may not be recognised as such because the rapid sequence of chronological events might not yet be evident. The temporal development of the nervous system of a child may actually outstrip the opposing effect of a disease process. A child with even a fatally progressive muscular dystrophy may for a time appear to be improving. The onset of dementia in a child may be particularly insidious because the retarding effect of the pathological process may at first do no more than to keep pace with normal intellectual development. It is only through a sound knowledge of the developmental timetable that the paediatric neurologist or the paediatrician is able to make an early diagnosis in such cases, and then usually with the aid of psychometric testing at intervals by an experienced operator.

Defects of motor function in mid and late childhood are summarised below and subsequently discussed in detail. Those causing death in early life are excluded from the list as they are not relevant to the consideration of 'The Clumsy Child'.

1. *Progressive*
   a. Neoplastic:
      Frontal—weakness, spasticity and frontal ataxia
      Parietal—sensory ataxia, parietal ataxia, apraxia and Gerstmann's syndrome
      Cerebellar—ataxia and dysequilibrium
      Spinal cord—weakness and spasticity.
   b. Metabolic:
      Poisoning by external agents—lead, mercury and DDT
      Drug toxicity—anticonvulsants, sedatives and tranquillisers
      Aminoacidurias—Hartnup disease, argininosuccinicaciduria and phenylketonuria
      Leucodystrophies—metachromatic leucodystrophy and Pelizaeus Merzbacher disease (they occur in the relevant age groups under discussion)
      Lipid storage disease—atypical forms, Spielmeyer–Vogt disease occurring in this relevant age group
      Wilson's disease with abnormal movements
      Hepatic pre-coma—with choreiform movements and 'asterixis' (liver flap).
   c. Degenerative:
      Heredofamilial spinocerebellar degenerations including Friedreich's ataxia, Marie's ataxia and Roussy–Levy syndrome
      Other cerebellar syndromes—ataxia telangiectasia, Fahr's disease, a-beta-lipoproteinaemia (Bassen–Kornzweig disease)
      Extrapyramidal syndromes—Huntington's chorea, juvenile paralysis agitans, Hallervorden–Spatz disease, rheumatic chorea
      Spinal and brainstem disorders—Syringomyelia, Arnold–Chiari malformation.
   d. Neuromuscular diseases:
      Kugelberg–Welander disease
      Peripheral nervous system disorders
      i. acquired polyneuropathy, e.g. metabolic, post-infective, vitamin deficiency and toxic

    ii. hereditary neuropathy, e.g. Déjérine–Sottas disease (hypertrophic polyneuritis), Charcot–Marie–Tooth disease (peroneal muscular atrophy), Refsum's disease (heredopathia atactica poly-neuritiformis), Tangier disease (a-alpha-lipoproteinaemia)

Progressive muscular dystrophy, especially Duchenne dystrophy

Polymyositis

Benign congenital myopathy—e.g. central core disease, megaconial myopathy, nemaline myopathy

Myotonia congenita

Myasthenia gravis.

  e. Miscellaneous:

Hydrocephalus which affects motor function particularly in the lower limbs

Myoclonic epilepsy—especially progressive diseases such as Unverricht–Lundborg disease and subacute sclerosing pan-encephalitis

Acute cerebellar ataxia (cerebellar form of acute disseminated encephalomyelitis)

Demyelinative disease—Schilder's disease and multiple sclerosis.

2. *Non-progressive*

  a. Congenital encephalopathies—comprise the largest group including all cases most often designated 'cerebral palsy'.

  b. Minimal cerebral dysfunction.

  c. Sequelae of acquired brain injury:

Post-traumatic

Post-meningitic

Post-encephalitic

Vascular accidents

Anoxia

Hypoglycaemia.

  d. Psychiatric disorders and mental defects:

Simple tics

Compound tics (Gilles de la Tourette syndrome)

Choreiform syndrome

Mental retardation.

  e. Miscellaneous:

Visual defects (visual failure, squint, congenital nystagmus)

Arthropathies (traumatic, rheumatoid, arthrogryposis)

Orthopaedic problems

Aural vertigo (Ménière's disease and benign intermittent vertigo of children).

Progressive Motor Defects in Children

Neoplasm

The natural history of cerebral tumour is such that eventually all cases will result in disturbances of motor function. With surgical intervention and other methods of treatment, cure or palliation may usually be effected. Because tumours of the frontal lobe may affect the precentral gyrus or motor cortex and its subcortical connections there may be an early appearance of contralateral weakness and spasticity. A more subtle disturbance of motor function occurs with tumour occupation of the prefrontal region of the brain giving rise to a general slowness of affect and of movement. This slowness or abulia coupled with the classical disinhibited behaviour pattern observed in frontal lobe disease may be wrongly attributed to malevolent emotional influences. The frequent complicating feature of epilepsy, either generalised or Jacksonian in type, or of motor aphasia immediately discloses the organic nature of such a presentation. Tremor of the type encountered in either paralysis agitans or cerebellar disease is occasionally observed and is not infrequently ipsilateral. Ataxia resembling that of cerebellar disease may develop and may reflect involvement of the fronto-ponto-cerebellar neural system although the origin of the ataxia found under these circumstances is unclear (Alpers and Mancall, 1971). Temporal and occipital lobe tumours do not produce effects on the motor system until advanced when there may be secondary pressure effects upon motor pathways.

Parietal lobe tumours may result in ataxia as a result of disturbance of cortical sensory mechanisms. Inco-ordination of motor function may occur purely as the result of a loss of input of sensory information (sensory ataxia). The true nature of the movement disorder may only become evident when the child exhibits astereognosis or loss of joint position sense or two-point discrimination, for superficial sensory modalities may be intact. Pseudoathetotic movements, aggravated by closing the eyes, may be observed in the contralateral limb as the result of deafferentation. Apraxia in its classical forms appears in lesions of both dominant and non-dominant parietal lobes. The subject may exhibit constructional apraxia, usually associated with dressing apraxia where there is an inability to appreciate shape and form such as the configuration of clothing. Writing, drawing, constructional tasks and dressing become either awkward or impossible. Destruction of the postero-inferior part of the dominant parietal lobe may be characterised by right–left disorientation, finger agnosia, agraphia and acalculia—the components of Gerstmann's syndrome. Disorders of the body scheme with inattention or neglect of one half may be encountered. Apraxias of motor, ideomotor and ideational type may be a feature of parietal and frontal lobe tumours, especially with corpus callosum or bilateral involvement implying widespread disease.

Of all intracranial neoplasms, cerebellar tumours are the most common in childhood. They also produce the most profound disintegration of movement. Intrinsic impairment of cerebellar function may be compounded by the secondary effects of raised intracranial pressure in producing cerebellar ataxia. The non-specific effect of producing obstructive hydrocephalus with an enlarging fourth ventricle may result in compression of the superior cerebellar peduncles. Midline tumours affecting the cerebellar vermis are more likely to result in ataxia of gait and speech, whereas more laterally disposed tumours in the cerebellar hemisphere will usually cause an ipsilateral ataxia of the upper and lower limbs with characteristic intention tremor.

Spinal tumours may produce ataxia, particularly when infiltrating or compressing the cervical spinal cord in the region of the foramen magnum and spreading into the posterior fossa. However, an ataxia of gait may be a prominent early feature of an even more caudally placed spinal cord tumour when there is an otherwise subtle clinical involvement of either the posterior or lateral columns on routine physical examination.

Metabolic disease

With increasing knowledge, particularly in the field of neurochemistry, the list of metabolic disorders enlarges at the expense of those previously relegated to degenerative or idiopathic categories. In patients with acute metabolic disturbance there is often an associated clouding of consciousness. More chronic or insidious involvement of the central nervous system is more likely to be confused with neurodevelopmental dysfunction because there may be no lateralisation of symptomatology. As with developmental syndromes of cerebral dysfunction, there tends to be a diffuse rather than circumscribed abnormality of the brain. This parallel provides a rationale for the assumption that neurodevelopmental dysfunction may well have a metabolic basis for the impairment of brain function in a primarily physiological rather than anatomical sense.

Most instances of lead poisoning are due to chronic exposure and the illness often has an insidious onset. Although the mode of entry in the younger child is usually by ingestion, in older subjects there may be exposure by inhalation or rarely by absorption through the skin. The child may show motor regression with loss of skilled movements as well as ataxia, muscular weakness or paralysis. In chronic mercurial poisoning the neurological symptoms include a coarse shaking tremor superimposed on a finer background tremor and cerebellar ataxia. Minamata disease due to mercurial pollution of seawater in southern Japan affected predominantly children under the age of 10 years. Its manifestations included dysarthria, truncal and limb ataxia and intention and resting tremor, with similar involvement of affected animals. Other heavy metals including thallium and arsenic and certain organic toxins in insecticides exert their deleterious effect on the motor system by damaging peripheral nerves.

Drug toxicity is a very potent cause of ataxia at all ages. In paediatric age groups the neurotoxic effects of anticonvulsant, tranquilliser and sedative medication are of considerable practical importance in the context of defects of motor function. The drugs which are most often prescribed for children with neuropsychiatric disorders may indeed vitiate the prime clinical features for which they have been prescribed. In the case of diphenylhydantoin (Dilantin, Epanutin) ataxia may appear quite insidiously, long after there has been an apparent stabilisation of dosage. Variability of absorption of the drug may be complicated further by variations in its transport with the concurrent administration of other anticonvulsants such as carbamazepine (Tegretol), barbiturates and sulthiame (Ospolot). The capricious side effects of diphenylhydantoin are well appreciated by the neurologist and the paediatrician, but the occasional supervention of ataxia may escape unnoticed. The clinician may also be slow to recognise the relevance of drug toxicity in most cases where there is no associated drowsiness. Thus for a period of weeks or months the child might easily be assumed incorrectly to be naturally clumsy. Occasionally the associated features of vomiting, dysarthria, nystagmus and ataxia may wrongly alert the clinician to the possibility of an underlying progressive neurological disorder. The occurrence of diphenylhydantoin toxicity might be greatly reduced if the attending clinician were always to check for the presence of nystagmus which is an early indicator of overmedication. Monitoring plasma drug levels by the newer methods of gas chromatography is likely to lead to more efficacious treatment. Very occasionally, diphenylhydantoin may cause irreversible damage of cerebellar function. Barbiturates and carbamazepine are more likely to result in drowsiness or hyperactive behaviour than nystagmus and ataxia in children, but the latter features certainly may occur.

Sedative medication in children does not produce ataxia except in moderate or large dosage, but in these cases it is seldom of practical diagnostic importance as ataxia virtually always should be anticipated. Tranquilliser medication with phenothiazines and related compounds may be a potent cause of motor dysfunction. Even when employed in small dosage, many clinicians prefer to anticipate the possible extrapyramidal side-effects of haloperidol in particular by prescribing anti-Parkinsonian drugs such as benztropine. When phenothiazine drugs exert their influence on the extrapyramidal system and produce such dramatic effects as spasmodic torticollis, retrocollis, and oculogyric crises, the causal relationship is unmistakable. Sometimes the alteration of tone or the production of athetoid or tremulous movement may disturb neurological function more subtly and the net effect may be accepted as an integral part of the neuropsychiatric syndrome under treatment. Drugs of the tricyclic group often are employed in the treatment of nocturnal enuresis, and more occasionally for hyperkinesia and depressive problems in children. It should not be overlooked that these and other psychotropic medications may occasionally result in mild tremor and other extrapyramidal symptoms which could give rise to unnecessary added anxiety.

In children of school age, Hartnup disease is probably the only disorder of amino-acid metabolism which might produce ataxia. Clinically the disorder is episodic and associated with other features of pellagra including rash, diarrhoea and psychosis. Ataxia and nystagmus may be observed. Patients with urea cycle disorders may exhibit intermittent ataxia corresponding to periods of ammonia intoxication precipitated by protein loading in the diet or intercurrent infection. Mental deficiency and early death are the rule in other aminoacidurias which affect motor function.

Although metachromatic leucodystrophy usually has its onset in early childhood, cases with a more chronic course may occur in late childhood. Amongst clinical manifestations affecting the motor system there may be cerebellar abnormalities including ataxia, nystagmus and tremor. Involvement of the peripheral nervous system contributes to the disturbance of motor function. Another leucodystrophy which may manifest motor dysfunction in mid or later childhood is Pelizaeus–Merzbacher disease, a sex-linked recessively inherited condition with the early appearance of cerebellar signs including ataxia, action tremor and dysarthria. The precise nature of sudanophilic leucodystrophy is controversial, but cases may arise in late childhood or adulthood, affecting both sexes and otherwise having a superficial resemblance to the clinical characteristics of Pelizaeus Merzbacher disease. As other leucodystrophies result in death in infancy they are not a practical consideration here.

The distinctive feature of motor dysfunction in hepatic enccphalopathy is the so-called 'liver flap' or asterixis. This coarse, flapping tremor has been ascribed to the intermittent loss of sustained muscular contraction necessary for the maintenance of postural fixation. Repeated grimacing and other athetoid features, especially affecting the hands, may manifest together with motor restlessness and twitching. Usually other features of advanced liver failure including severe jaundice and drowsiness are evident. Wilson's disease (hepatolenticular degeneration) may present with hepatic dysfunction which also is often the cause of final demise. The condition usually has a neurological presentation from mid childhood to adolescence where hand tremor and ataxia of gait are early features. Protean forms of abnormal movement vary from choreoathetosis and dystonia in some patients to cerebellar signs associated with Parkinsonism in others.

Lipid storage diseases usually do not present as disorders of the motor system as their most characteristic features are progressive visual and intellectual deterioration. However, in most cases with delayed onset in childhood and adolescence there may be a predominantly 'cerebellar' type of presentation.

Degenerative disorders

Advances in clinical neurology usually refer to the elucidation of underlying disease processes, and to more sophisticated management of neurological problems. Occasionally when new neurological syndromes are described they tend to lie within the category of the degenerative disorders. Despite this tendency, the list of degenerative disorders is probably diminishing pari passu with the disclosure of enzymatic and virological bases for a number of neuropathological processes hitherto ascribed to idiopathic degenerative causes. There remains, however, a very hard core of abiotrophic processes which at present defy precise aetiological classification. In some instances, an hereditary factor is of prime importance, and in others there are observable biochemical phenomena which are basically epiphenomenological rather than aetiological. It is implicit that diseases which fall into this category are incurable, but eugenic counselling plays a very important preventative role in conditions of heritable nature.

The most familiar form of heredofamilial spinocerebellar degeneration of childhood is Friedreich's ataxia. The onset is usually very insidious, and a history may be obtained that the child was slow to walk and always clumsy, although normal early development is usual. The presenting symptoms are unsteadiness of gait, difficulty with games and general manual indexterity. Overt signs of cerebellar dysfunction, such as nystagmus, or intention tremor of the upper limbs and disturbance of posterior column function contributing to the entire problem of ataxia, are later features. Cerebellar dysarthria and later weakness of the lower limbs may appear. Important associated features of cardiomyopathy, scoliosis and pes cavus may be evident from the outset. In the earlier stages of the disorder in mid childhood, the differential diagnosis might well include the clumsy child syndrome or other disorders of cerebellar function.

There are many other variants of the hereditary spinocerebellar ataxias. These include hereditary spastic paraplegia where attention is first attracted to the child on account of its stiff and clumsy gait, and the Roussy—Levy syndrome in which there is an overlap of the manifestations of Friedreich's ataxia and peroneal muscular atrophy. Sanger—Brown's and Marie's ataxias may commence in adolescence and differ largely from Friedreich's ataxia in the existence of ocular manifestations including optic atrophy and ophthalmoplegia.

There are a number of other progressive cerebellar syndromes, usually of hereditary nature but more diverse in their clinicopathological manifestations than the foregoing group. These include ataxia telangiectasia (Louis—Bar syndrome) characterised by the early onset of cerebellar ataxia and the presence of telangiectases in the conjunctivae and skin creases. Choreoathetosis may be present in some patients and the speech is dysarthric. Recurrent infections are the rule and substantive support for the diagnosis may be obtained by noting absent or low serum gamma 1A globulin. The Bassen—Kornzweig syndrome presents in early childhood with symptoms of malabsorption and progressive cerebellar ataxia. A-beta-lipoproteinaemia in the serum and acanthocytosis in the blood film substantiate the diagnosis.

Huntington's chorea may arise in early childhood, but, unlike the far commoner adult cases, muscular rigidity and occasionally cerebellar ataxia are the more usual defects of motor function. Also in most juvenile cases epilepsy is characteristic and dementia universal, but the potentially difficult clinical diagnosis is simplified by the autosomal dominant pattern of inheritance. Disorders of the basal ganglia in children are extremely rare. Dystonia musculorum deformans (torsion dystonia) usually commences between the ages of five and 15 years, and in most cases involuntary movements begin first in one foot with intermittent plantar flexion and inversion at the ankle. Early diagnosis is difficult without a positive family history, but it is an important consideration because of the onset with gait disorder.

Other rare familial degenerative disorders of the corpus striatum in childhood include Hallervorden—Spatz disease, where rigidity and athetosis of the limbs may present in middle childhood, and juvenile paralysis agitans which is characterised by rhythmic resting tremor diminished by volitional movement.

Disturbances of the neuraxis at spinal and brainstem level include both syringomyelia and the Arnold—Chiari malformation. These two conditions which are probably pathogenetically interrelated may both cause compromise of corticospinal tract function with a resultant defect of movement particularly in the lower limbs. Ataxia may result either from sensory impairment or disturbance of cerebellar function.

Neuromuscular diseases

Progressive spinal muscular atrophy of Kugelberg Welander type exhibits a wide variability of age of onset and rate of progress. The subject, usually in early life, exhibits a very slowly progressive wasting and weakness of muscles with hypotonia and other features of lower motor neurone involvement. Its differentiation from progressive muscular dystrophy may not be possible on purely clinical grounds and may require diagnostic support from electromyography, nerve conduction studies, serum enzyme estimations, and histological and histochemical studies. Previously patients in this category were frequently misdiagnosed as suffering from limb girdle muscular dystrophy.

Polyneuropathy is a relatively uncommon occurrence in children. In cases of toxic and metabolic origin the presentation is either acute or subacute. The nature of the Guillain–Barré syndrome can usually be distinguished because of its subacute onset, its tendency to follow in the wake of exanthemata or banal upper respiratory tract infection and the not infrequent involvement both of cranial nerve and respiratory musculature. Much more germane to the issue of clumsiness in children are the rare hereditary neuropathies of Déjérine–Sottas disease (hypertrophic polyneuritis) and Refsum's disease (heredopathia atactica polyneuritiformis).

In some cases of the former condition there is a close clinical resemblance to Charcot–Marie–Tooth disease (peroneal muscular atrophy) with which it still has a somewhat uncertain interrelationship. Although sensory symptoms are usually prominent in the early stages, difficulty in walking is often an early complaint. Tangier disease (a-alpha-lipoproteinaemia) is a hereditary disorder of lipid metabolism distinguished by an almost complete absence of high-density plasma lipoproteins, reduction of other plasma lipids and visceromegaly due to storage of cholesterol esters. Retinitis pigmentosa and peripheral neuropathy have been observed.

Of all the myopathic disorders in children, none produces a more characteristic disturbance of motor function that progressive muscular dystrophy of the Duchenne type. Its transmission as a sex-linked recessive characteristic results in its almost invariable manifestation in males with transmission through unaffected females. The earliest symptom usually is clumsiness in walking with a tendency to fall. First attempts to walk are often delayed or awkward, and the inability to run is an early feature. Later, with difficulty observed in climbing stairs, and in rising from the floor and the characteristic method of climbing up the legs to reach a standing position (Gowers' sign), the diagnosis of a progressive disorder becomes evident. The waddling gait, protuberant abdomen and weakness of the limbs are more advanced features and loss of ambulation usually occurs by the eleventh year.

Polymyositis in childhood is usually associated with skin involvement (dermatomyositis). It produces considerable constitutional upset including fever, oedema and abdominal pain; weakness of the extremities commencing in the upper limbs is characteristic. A disturbance of deglutition in the earlier stages is often encountered. Differentiation from Duchenne muscular dystrophy is not always easy, and even muscle biopsy may yield equivocal results. Of great practical importance is the responsiveness of polymyositis to corticosteroid therapy.

There are a number of relatively benign congenital myopathies which have been delineated by histological, histochemical and ultrastructural studies. These include central core disease, nemaline, megaconial, pleoconial and myotubular myopathy. In general these patients have shown varying degrees of proximal muscular wasting and weakness often of slowly progressive or almost non-progressive nature. Type I and Type II muscle fibre hypoplasia can probably be added to this group where some patients exhibiting muscle weakness in childhood have shown slowness in achieving motor milestones and general clumsiness of gait and movement attributable to muscular weakness.

Benign congenital hypotonia, a term devised by Walton (1956) for children with delayed motor control and muscular hypotonia in infancy, represents a heterogenous group of myopathic disorders which may include some of the above-named categories. The condition probably comprises an heterogenous group of cases of benign nature where in many instances the children outgrow their disorder. Weakness and hypotonia is associated with delay in the acquisition of motor milestones and general inferiority in motor activity.

Families of patients with dystrophia myotonica not infrequently include affected young children. The relatively high incidence of mental deficiency in this group allows for lesser compensation of the impaired control of movement. The children usually manifest a considerable weakness of facial musculature as well as more distal involvement of limb muscles. The difficulty of relaxation of muscles after contraction (myotonia), particularly involving the handgrips, may sometimes result in considerable awkwardness, and may respond to treatment with muscle membrane stabilisers such as quinine sulphate and procainamide. The characteristic stiff, stumbling gait on first attempting to walk after resting in patients with myotonia congenita (Thomsen's disease) clearly distinguishes this disorder from the other myotonias of childhood. Variable weakness and excessive muscle fatiguability are the hallmarks of myasthenia gravis.

Miscellaneous

Because of the obvious clinical feature of an abnormally enlarging cranium, children with overt congenital hydrocephalus do not really present any serious diagnostic problem. Communicating and non-communicating hydrocephalus result in an accumulation of cerebrospinal fluid pressure due to obstruction of its circulation and absorption. During its evolution the hydrocephalus sometimes may become compensated because of the establishment of an equilibrium between the rates of cerebrospinal fluid absorption and production. A state of decompensation may occur later in life, occasionally as the result of minor head trauma, and if the cranial sutures are fused and cranial enlargement cannot occur a sharp rise of intracranial pressure may result. Acquired hydrocephalus results from lesions which block cerebrospinal fluid circulation, such as tumours within the ventricular system or in the posterior fossa, or lesions which interfere with absorption, such as meningitis or subarachnoid haemorrhage. An insidious onset of hydrocephalus may produce an abnormality of gait as an initial symptom because of the production of either diplegia or cerebellar ataxia. The latter results from pressure on the superior cerebellar peduncles from enlargement of the fourth ventricle. Yakovlev (1947) has explained the propensity of hydrocephalus to produce diplegia in that the longer course of the corticospinal fibres subserving motor function to the lower limbs and their closer apposition to the enlarging lateral ventricles renders them more vulnerable to the effects of compression. In any child showing differentially greater motor impairment of the lower rather than the upper limbs, borderline enlargement of the cranium may be a valuable contributory physical sign which may alert one to the possibility of an underlying hydrocephalic process. Although compensated hydrocephalus might be diagnosable definitively with air contrast ventricular studies, such investigatory procedures are usually injudicious as they may precipitate a state of decompensation which could require emergency operative intervention. In some cases, treatment with acetazolamide, frusemide or dexamethasone might reduce intracranial tension until the hydrocephalus resolves spontaneously once again.

Patients with myoclonic epilepsy certainly may give the impression of undue clumsiness. Subjects who suffer from varying forms of idiopathic epilepsy often will manifest myoclonic jerks particularly involving the upper extremities, especially when first arising in the mornings presumably before anticonvulsant medication has taken full effect. The child may unwittingly drop or fling objects from the hand and prove a source of annoyance particularly when eating at the breakfast table. Progressive myoclonus epilepsy (Unverricht–Lundborg disease) is characterised by a late childhood onset of convulsive seizures and the subsequent development of myoclonus before the onset of dementia, rigidity and death in early adulthood. Myoclonus often first appears in the upper extremities before gradually becoming generalised. Eating, writing, dressing and walking may become greatly impaired and speech may be interrupted by jerky vocalisations. The rhythmical onset of myoclonic jerking often confined to one area of the body might antedate the onset of dementia in children suffering from subacute sclerosing pan-encephalitis. These two conditions included among the so-called 'myoclonic dementias' are only diagnostically problematical in their earlier stages.

Demyelinative disorders in children are usually of acute or subacute nature. The commonest form of post-infective encephalitis (acute disseminated encephalomyelitis) is a multifocal involvement principally of brainstem structures. There is usually widespread cranial nerve, motor and sensory impairment. Although acute cerebellar ataxia of childhood is often considered in a separate category, it probably represents a pure cerebellar form of acute disseminated encephalomyelitis which tends to have a more benign course with recovery over several weeks. Multiple sclerosis, a rare entity in children, has protean manifestations where profound disorders of motor function arise from destructive plaques within the corticospinal and cerebellar pathways. Schilder's disease is probably more accurately considered with the demyelinative rather than with the leucodystrophic disorders. Although the condition may at first involve corticospinal pathways, it is usual for this asymmetrical hemispheric disease to result in visual and mental changes in the earlier stages. Its characteristic episodic progression differentiates it from most of the degenerative disorders.

Non-progressive Motor Defects in Children

Congenital encephalopathies

These comprise the largest non-progressive group, which is most often designated 'cerebral palsy'. Although anoxic birth injury has been implicated as the fundamental aetiological factor in a large proportion of patients with cerebral palsy, there must also be a considerable number which are due to cerebral maldevelopment. Anoxic birth injury may result from circumstances concerned with pre-eclampsia, antepartum haemorrhage, prolonged labour and abnormal delivery including forceps, breech and caesarian extractions. Hypermyelination of the basal ganglia known as status marmoratus can be correlated with anoxic birth injury on the one hand and the presence of choreoathetosis and diplegia on the other. Fetal and perinatal cerebral infarction resulting from occlusions, usually in internal carotid artery territory, may result in unilateral porencephaly. Symmetrical porencephalic malformation of the brain more usually has a developmental origin. Intracranial bleeding may result from the tearing of dural sinuses with the production of either a subdural or intracerebral haematoma.

Congenital malformations of the brain which may take on many forms may be induced by noxious agents, but causal factors often cannot be delineated. Pathological findings include ectopias of grey matter and large variations in thickness of the grey cortical ribbon. There may be a simplification or overcomplication of the configuration of the gyral pattern of the cerebral cortex. Certain structures such as the corpus callosum or the cerebellum may be either absent or vestigial.

Varying aetiological agents resulting in intra-uterine cerebral maldevelopment, often with encephaloclasis, are listed as follows:

1. Maternal infections including rubella, cytomegalic inclusion body disease, toxoplasmosis and syphilis
2. Maternal diabetes
3. Maternal drug ingestion including teratogenic toxins, metabolic antagonists and milder non-specific factors from cigarette smoking
4. Fetal irradiation
5. Vitamin deficiencies
6. Chromosomal anomalies
7. Kernicterus usually related to Rh incompatability producing haemorrhagic disease of the newborn.

The essential overt features of so-called 'cerebral palsy' include: (1) weakness; (2) spasticity; and (3) abnormal movements.

These features usually manifest earlier than the motor dysfunctions which are characteristic of the specific 'clumsy child' syndrome. The severest cases of congenital encephalopathy present in early infancy whereas milder affections may be apparent only to parents or medical advisors when there is a significant delay in motor milestones. There are obviously all gradations of cerebral palsy in which the most serious cases exhibit profound mental retardation, quadriplegia and epilepsy or sometimes profound dysarthria with double athetosis. The mildest cases are those of normally intelligent children without symptoms, but with physical signs such as extensor plantar responses or asymmetrical deep tendon reflexes. The most obvious features of patients with cerebral palsy, apart from inconstant factors such as epilepsy and mental retardation, are defects of the motor system. In the last few decades there has been an increasing awareness of the associated problems of sensory disturbance and perceptuo-motor dysfunction. These latter disturbances contribute to the total problem of ungainly motor activity. Their importance lies mainly in the province of rehabilitation because the development of physical skills in these children is partly contingent upon their perceptive abilities.

The therapist must take cognisance of the fact that the development of visuomotor and sensory skills requires a different approach from the facilitation of motor function in a child beset by spasticity, weakness or abnormal movements. When a child is unable to cope with the normal school environment because of his physical disabilities he is probably best treated at a cerebral palsy centre. In these centres provision is made not only for the formal education of the child, but also for a parallel programme of therapy directed towards physical rehabilitation. Schoolteachers work side by side with physiotherapists, speech therapists, occupational therapists and social workers. Their efforts are integrated usually by a physician specially qualified in the field of cerebral palsy. Unfortunately a final integration of these children into the mainstream of adult endeavour is not always possible and occupation in sheltered workshops may be the only reasonable final alternative. In less severely afflicted individuals, it may be possible to effect final integration into the community at large, but this sometimes requires special consideration from sympathetic employers. Less severely afflicted children such as those with mild but obvious congenital hemiplegias, athetosis and ataxic cerebral palsy usually attend normal schools, where often they have much the same potential as their peers. Children with very mild motor manifestations of cerebral palsy, but with visuospatial defects, may be paradoxically even more disadvantaged because of the lack of recognition of their problems by parents and teachers. Minimal degrees of weakness, spasticity or ataxia may be misconstrued as strong contralateral handedness. Presumably hemiplegic cerebral palsy occurs at approximately equal frequency on left and right sides of the body. For every one child who becomes obligatorily rather than constitutionally right-handed because of minimal left hemiparesis there must be a child who becomes obligatorily left-handed because of minimal right hemiparesis. The obligate dextral is more likely to escape notice than the obligate sinistral because people are mindful of the higher incidence of congenital encephalopathy in left-handers. Hence, because the total number of sinistral children is much less than that of dextrals, the proportion of sinistrals with minimal hemiparesis is much higher than that of dextrals.

Although a careful neurological examination of children with minimal cerebral palsy will elicit physical signs, a large proportion of these children who attend normal schools very possibly go through life without knowing of their disadvantage. Perhaps they may be aware of only minor inconveniences such as asymmetry of the feet when buying shoes. Curiously they may be even somewhat advantaged by the exhibition of ambidexterity (ambilevity) where tools and utensils may be used with equal facility on either side, but never as well as by the normal individual with a well-developed cerebral dominance. Ambidexterity in this context is a misnomer because the individual might be regarded as having two 'minor' rather than two 'major' hemispheres for manual dominance. Hence, employment of the term ambilevity is probably more appropriate.

Minimal cerebral dysfunction

A large, hitherto neglected subgroup of congenital encephalopathies, entitled minimal cerebral dysfunction, is now rightfully receiving worldwide interest and attention. This category includes children with significant impairments of motor or intellectual functions with *minimal,* or absence of, conventional neurological signs. However, the term minimal is unsatisfactory because it refers to a dearth of neurological physical signs, whereas the dysfunction may be moderate, severe or even *maximal.*

There is an obvious clinical overlap between patients suffering from classical cerebral palsy syndromes and those in the category of so-called minimal cerebral dysfunction. The hallmark of cerebral palsy is congenital motor dysfunction associated with conventional signs elicited by routine neurological examination. Paradoxically, the child with no conventional neurological signs may manifest defects of motor functioning of greater personal impact than cerebral palsy and which interfere more profoundly with the functions of learning and performance. It is very probable that many cases of minimal cerebral dysfunction are variants of congenital encephalopathy in the structural organic sense. Where on the one hand a circumscribed area of neurological damage or maldevelopment may give rise to spasticity, abnormal movements or weakness, a comparable organic condition on the other hand may affect other parameters of neurological function of similar or even greater moment.

Often the patient with overt cerebral palsy will also manifest conditions which are usually included in the syndrome of minimal cerebral dysfunction. However, a structural organic aetiology is not always implied. Apparent abnormalities in some cases are probably variations from the norm, and the changes become less obvious with maturation. In many if not most cases, the dysfunction probably has no truly organic substrate. The child in these instances probably functions normally with respect to its own central nervous system, but subnormally in comparison to the central nervous system of other children within the same age group and environment.

Children with specific learning disabilities, especially with visuomotor impairment, have often been considered as belonging to the group of minimal cerebral dysfunction. There are some who would equate the terms specific learning disability and minimal cerebral dysfunction. Obviously there is a very large area of overlap between these two broad categories which, however, are not strictly comparable, as the former refers to an educational concept and the latter to a neurological one. Both terms refer to disordered higher mental functions, especially to specific deficiencies in certain areas of intellectual functioning where the majority of the intellect is preserved. In contrast, cerebral palsy more specifically refers to various parameters of motor dysfunction. A more detailed discussion of minimal cerebral dysfunction is deferred until later in this chapter.

Sequelae of acquired brain injury

Nothing can be more devastating in its effect on a child than severe cerebral trauma. Nevertheless it is remarkable how frequently total or near-total recovery can occur after apparent catastrophic brain injury. Conversely, it may be wise for the clinician to be guarded in his prognosis in children who have had a cerebral contusion or laceration when there is initial rapid improvement, as minor disabilities in the field of behaviour disorders and learning disabilities may linger. Post-traumatic epilepsy is more likely to supervene when contiguous meningeal and cerebral cortical disruption results in the formation of a meningocerebral cicatrix. The irritant epileptogenic properties of such a cerebral scar may be an isolated post-traumatic effect where the subject does not show any further manifestations of the previous cerebral injury.

Both meningitis and encephalitis may cause severe permanent neurological deficit, and rapid recovery from the acute infection unfortunately does not always imply eventual total recovery. Quite apart from the very frequent behaviour disorders observed in these groups, epilepsy and mild cerebral dysfunction in varying intellectual areas may persist.

Amongst the group of encephalitic or post-encephalitic disorders the condition of rheumatic chorea (Sydenham's chorea) might conveniently be considered here. Known also as chorea minor, the condition may occur after antecedent rheumatic fever and may be a manifestation of a hypersensitivity reaction following streptococcus Group A infection. The child characteristically exhibits spontaneous movements of choreoathetoid type involving face and limbs. Voluntary movements are interrupted by jerky involuntary motor activity which is frequently more prominent on one side of the body than on the other. The child may lose clarity of speech. Inco-ordination of the limbs is usually associated with varying degrees of weakness and results in tremendous clumsiness of performance profoundly affecting everyday activities such as handwriting and eating. Minor degrees of chorea minor may be difficult to differentiate from psychogenic tic. However, the condition is usually recognised and probably tends to be overdiagnosed in cases of the choreiform syndrome of Prechtl and Stemmer (1962).

Cerebrovascular disease of children is rather more aetiologically elusive than in adults where atheroma is usually implicated. It has been postulated (Bickerstaff, 1964) that the acute hemiplegic syndrome of childhood is due to an endarteritis and thrombosis of the internal carotid artery resulting from contiguous spread of the inflammatory process in patients with pharyngitis and tonsillitis. More occasionally acute hemiplegic syndromes in infancy and childhood are due to occlusion of the middle cerebral arterial trunk. Sometimes recovery is rapid and complete, but occasionally the patients are left with lifelong hemiplegia. In these children there is an inherent similarity to congenital hemiplegia, with underdevelopment of the affected limbs, except that athetosis is less likely to occur.

Of all the organs, the brain is the most sensitive to temporary reduction of blood oxygen tension. Anoxic brain injury may result from insufficient oxygen reaching the arterial blood either due to defective pulmonary ventilation or reduced atmospheric oxygen tension. In cases of severe anaemia due to haemorrhage or inactivation of haemoglobin by carbon monoxide poisoning, less oxygen is transported to cerebral tissue. Failure of the circulation with stagnation of blood also results in reduced transport of oxygen and its defective utilisation by tissue cells may also occur in toxic states. A single severe hypoxic episode causes diffuse damage to the cerebral and cerebellar cortices and to a lesser extent the globus pallidus and other subcortical grey structures. The pyramidal cells in the Sommer's sector of the hippocampus, and the Purkinje cells of the cerebellum, are selectively more vulnerable than other neurones. The lesions of hypoxic encephalopathy in the neonate consist of foci of usually symmetrical tissue necrosis in the inferior colliculi and other brainstem nuclei rather than the cerebral cortex (Adams and Sidman, 1968). In hypoglycaemic encephalopathy there is also a special predilection for damage of cortical neurones and involvement of the basal ganglia and the hippocampus.

In more severe cases of anoxia or hypoglycaemia, patients who survive may remain unconscious in a state of decerebration or decortication. Less profound cerebral insult may result in varying degrees of dementia in association with cerebellar and extrapyramidal syndromes with ataxia, dysarthria and abnormal movements. It is assumed that anoxic brain injury is responsible for a large proportion of patients suffering from congenital encephalopathy with a wide range of manifestations including mental retardation, epilepsy, and pyramidal and extrapyramidal symptomatology.

Psychiatric disorders and mental defect

Perhaps the commonest disturbance of motor function of psychogenic origin is simple tic. The condition is characterised by the appearance of repetitive stereotyped movements which most commonly affect the facial muscles. The subject, usually a child under stress, may show repetitive eye blinking and facial grimacing, frequently accompanied by grunting-type vocalisations and shoulder shrugging. Occasionally the movements can be quite violent. They can always be suppressed, for at least a short period by an effort of will, but the subject soon succumbs by manifesting further stereotyped tics with renewed vigour. These spasmodic movements usually can be readily distinguished from choreiform movement in that the latter tends to be less stereotyped, more erratic and more difficult to control temporarily. There is usually no significant disturbance of physical performance in a child with psychogenic tic provided the tic frequency is not great enough to produce significant distraction from pursuing a physical act.

The syndrome of Gilles de la Tourette (maladie des tics) may be included in the category of psychogenic tic. It is characterised by motor inco-ordination accompanied by echolalia, palilalia and uncontrollable audible obscenities. Its onset is during childhood usually before the age of 10 years. Abnormal motor movements consisting of mild facial twitchings, blinking of the eyes or more severe jerkings of head and limbs are conspicious. There is a simultaneous profane utterance usually of a word concerning the sexual or excretory act. The condition is often progressive and it is possible that there may be an organic component in its aetiology. Haloperidol has been useful in controlling symptoms.

The choreiform syndrome of Prechtl and Stemmer (1962) almost certainly has a psychogenic component in many instances. In a series of children with learning difficulties, the distinct neurological syndrome could be identified in 50 cases. These children showed habitual clumsiness with choreiform movements. The large majority had a similar affection of the eye muscles leading to disturbances of conjugate movement, and difficulty in fixation and reading. There were specific difficulties in learning to read and write. Much of the clumsiness of children with the choreiform syndrome can be attributed to their extreme fidgetiness and increased motor restlessness. The condition probably represents a heightening of the physiological choreiform movements which are seen in all young children, especially below the age of seven years, and which are usually largely abolished by the age of 12 years. Serial physical examinations and observations on these children may show the choreiform movements to be much more in evidence on some occasions than on others. It is probable that the greatly variable performance in such instances might be influenced particularly by emotional factors. This type of choreiform movement might easily be mistaken for chorea minor, a factor of considerable importance with respect to management for the unfortunate child may be required unnecessarily to take a very protracted course of penicillin.

Mental handicap of any origin is a frequent cause of motor retardation and clumsiness. Many of the categories of central nervous system disease alluded to in this chapter are associated with mental deficiency. Although there are scores of described causes of mental deficiency, which has an incidence of approximately 3 per cent in children, a substantial proportion of all cases are unclassifiable. Hypotonia and motor retardation are frequently encountered as exemplified in Down's syndrome. Even when there are no demonstrable neurological signs, mentally retarded children in general are clumsier than normal children. There is a lack of development of praxis and gnosis but the terms apraxia or agnosia are no more applicable to their perceptuomotor retardation than aphasia to their lack of speech development. Nonetheless their lack of motor facility is comparable to children with isolated developmental apraxia and agnosia or in some cases of 'minimal cerebral dysfunction' where by definition the intellect is normal. At present, clumsiness might well be regarded as a relatively neglected feature in children with mental deficiency where the more important issue of social training has a very high priority in management.

Miscellaneous

Although it might be obvious that defective vision can result in clumsiness and untidy performance, it occasionally remains unrecognised until discovered at a routine medical check at school. Correction of relatively mild errors of refraction may have a salutary effect on performance at school, particularly if the defective vision is only one of a number of minor handicaps affecting the child. Although frequently omitted, it is essential to include a check of visual acuity as part of the routine physical assessment in children who often do not recognise visual failure as a symptom. Robbed of binocular vision, the child with a non-paralytic squint is unlikely to perform well in ball games. It should not only be the prerogative of the ophthalmologist to test for primary and secondary eye deviation in suspected latent squint with the 'cover test', but also that of every medical practitioner who deals with children where defective vision or squint is suspected.

Congenital nystagmus is an hereditary disorder often noticeable in infancy and invariably associated with defective vision, usually in association with errors of refraction. A characteristic feature is the presence of pendular nystagmus in the primary position of the eyes. Defective motor performance may occur only because of the influence of poor vision in such cases. Congenital oculomotor apraxia of Cogan is characterised by difficulty in lateral pursuit eye movement, necessitating movement of the head to one or the other side to find or follow objects in the lateral visual field. These children are said to be slow to walk and may show an ungainliness because of their inability to make quick turns with proper facility; they also have difficulty in reading.

Arthropathies and other congenital or acquired skeletal abnormalities in childhood such as arthrogryposis or sequelae of limb fractures may certainly result in awkward movements. It is not unusual for children with the insidious onset of juvenile arthropathy to be referred for neurological assessment because of clumsiness even when the arthropathy itself has been recognised. Congenital bone and joint disorders of the lower limbs may certainly result in limping and other abnormalities of gait and are not always immediately recognised as orthopaedic rather than neurological in origin. The clinician should always be mindful of the trophic influence of a congenital neurological disturbance, particularly of the cauda equina or lumbar spinal cord as in spinal dysraphism (James and Lassman, 1967), on the development of the lower limbs.

Disturbances of equilibrium may occur as an aftermath of toxic and infective disorders of the labyrinth. Intermittent acute labyrinthine dysfunction occurring in benign intermittent vertigo of childhood or, rarely, juvenile Ménière's syndrome can hardly be confused with primary disturbances of motor function. Children so afflicted manifest sudden acute distress from vertigo and ataxia. Bilateral toxic labyrinthine damage from streptomycin, after an initial period of adjustment, may produce disequilibrium only at times of greater challenge to the motor system such as when playing sport.

MINIMAL CEREBRAL DYSFUNCTION

The 1962 International Study Group in Oxford originally agreed on this term, which can be regarded as an extension of ideas propounded by Denhoff and Robinault (1960) in their treatise on cerebral palsy and related disorders. These authors, who were optimistic in their approach regarding remediation, believed that cerebral palsy was not a definitive entity in itself, but one aspect of a broader syndrome of cerebral dysfunction. The broader concept of cerebral palsy is partially embodied in their assertion that 'brain damage' is seldom confined to motor areas. In the same vein, Denhoff, Laufer and Holden (1959) recognised six categories amongst the syndromes of cerebral dysfunction which included: (1) neuromotor (cerebral palsy); (2) intellectual; (3) epilepsy; (4) vision and hearing; (5) behavioural; (6) perceptual.

They considered that there was evidence to suggest diencephalic dysfunction as well as cortical damage to the organic substratum. These authors also made a plea for the replacement of the terms 'brain damage' and 'brain-injured child'.

The concept of minimal cerebral dysfunction has been crystallised further into a definition by the Task Force organised by the National Institute of Neurological Diseases and Blindness which incorporated "children of near average, average or above average general intelligence with certain learning or behavioural disabilities ranging from mild to severe, which are associated with deviations of function of the central nervous system. These deviations may manifest themselves by various combinations of impairment in perception, conceptualisation, language, memory and control of attention, impulse or motor function" (Clements, 1966a). As mentioned earlier, the deviant function of the central nervous system may not be at all subtle in terms of the manifestations of the child's difficulties. The term 'subtle' is used advisedly as its real meaning here is probably the tenuous or evasive nature of physical signs in this condition.

Various authors have speculated upon the definitions and classifications of manifestations of minimal cerebral dysfunction. In a multidisciplinary diagnostic clinic for handicapped children, Clemmens (1961) evaluated 525 patients of whom 19 per cent had minimal cerebral dysfunction or minimal brain damage with intellectual subnormalities. The importance of an interdisciplinary effort towards management of these children was stressed. A diagnostic evaluation plan relying on subtests of the Wechsler Intelligence Scale for Children and equivocal neurological signs has been described by Clements and Peters (1962). These authors remarked how often the child was described as awkward or clumsy either in fine muscle performance or overall co-ordination or both. It is indeed remarkable how frequently there may be disparities between the efficacy of motor functioning in one area such as handwriting and another such as running or dancing. Paine (1962) suggested that there was a syndrome of minimal brain damage with subclinical affections in each of four areas which may be stated as motor, mental, sensory and convulsive. In these chronic brain syndromes, specific clumsiness was included in the first category (motor) which also included: (1) minor choreoathetosis or tremor; (2) isolated hyper-reflexia; and (3) excessive clumsiness.

Clements, Lehtinen and Lukens (1963) listed the outstanding characteristics associated with the syndrome of children with minimal brain injury in whom a few or many of the symptoms may appear in a given child as follows:

1. Normal or above average intelligence
2. Specific learning deficits
3. Perceptual-motor deficits
4. General co-ordination deficits
5. Hyperkinesis
6. Impulsivity
7. Emotional lability
8. Short attention span and/or distractibility
9. Equivocal or 'soft' neurological signs
10. Borderline abnormal or abnormal EEG.

Clements (1966b) had estimated that five to 20 per cent of the general school population could be included in the category of minimal brain dysfunction, a fact which is therefore of major importance in the entire health field and which invites multidisciplinary interest and concern. MacKeith (1963) attempted to reconcile the views of various authorities when defining the concept of minimal brain damage. The general consensus was that there were deficiencies in the usage of this term. Later, MacKeith (1968) was of the view that a child discovered to have a particular brain dysfunction should be placed in a general category, since a handicap of one system or function is so commonly accompanied by a handicap in another or in others. There is much merit in the view that overall function should be spelled out in the eight fields of motor function, vision, hearing, language, intelligence, drive and concentration, and emotional and social function. The term 'neuro-developmental disorder' was used to cover the child with developmental delay due to social deprivation equally with the one who has a hemiplegia which is 'organic' and a child with specific learning disorders whose origin is usually obscured. The heterogeneity of the group designated as suffering from minimal brain damage was one of the main reasons why that term largely had been discarded in keeping with recommendations of the 1962 Oxford International Study Group on Child Neurology (Bax and MacKeith, 1963).

There are many—especially those involved in the education of children—who prefer to highlight the major problem and use the term 'learning disabilities' (Gallagher et al, 1969). These authors, concerned with educational aspects, expressed the view that the overall term minimal brain dysfunction emphasised the fact that certain children, while not grossly impaired, exhibited limited deviations of intellect and behaviour of such a nature as to require special resources for their management and education. Only a small percentage of the affected children are at present receiving adequate services. Task Force II attempted to define learning disabilities in a universally acceptable fashion. Among the definitions proffered was "Children with learning disabilities are those (1) who have educationally significant discrepancies among their sensory-motor, perceptual, cognitive, academic or related developmental levels which interfere with the performance of educational tasks; (2) who may or may not show demonstrable deviation in central nervous system functioning; and (3) whose disabilities are not secondary to general mental retardation, sensory deprivation or obvious emotional disturbance" (Haring and Bateman, 1969).

A reference to 'clumsy children' by Brain and Walton (1969) neatly explains the term within the concept of minimal cerebral dysfunction. A review of scientific knowledge regarding the learning disabilities of children with minimal cerebral dysfunction is incorporated in the report of Task Force III (Chalfant and Scheffelin, 1969). Block (1971) makes further attempts at classification and simplification of cerebral dysfunctions.

The bases of many of these more modern concepts of minimal cerebral dysfunction were originally expounded in writings by Kramer and Pollnow (1932), Kahn and Cohen (1934) and Gesell and Amatruda (1947). Collectively these authors had described many characteristics. Amongst these have been the motor restlessness, total inability to concentrate and disturbances in development of speech with preservation of intellect in the hyperkinetic syndrome in childhood. A surplus of inner impulsion (organic driveness) was thought to occur in individuals because of defective brainstem organisation with reference to this same syndrome. Also described were minor defects of speech and motor functioning with unsteadiness and clumsiness in young children with histories suggestive of birth injury, but sometimes with distinct improvement to the point of the children appearing almost normal as they grew older.

The importance of the recognition of minimal cerebral palsy has been stressed by Köng (1963) who warns of the possibility of rejection by parents and school teachers. Far from being a minimal problem, there often turned out to be a greater problem than was evident in even severe cerebral palsy. In 20 of her cases there were minimal physical signs of the usual neurological syndromes such as spasticity and athetosis. The inferiority complex in these children in some ways had been compensated for by nonsensical behaviour. The importance of early diagnosis lay in the fact that the children otherwise found great difficulty in coping with their environmental circumstances, apart from the attendant problems for parents and teachers. A simple explanation was said to give the child back a feeling of self respect and also to allow the parents to reappraise the management and handling of the child, with subsequent improvement of parent–child relationships (Wigglesworth, 1963). Early diagnosis and institution of treatment have been associated with better results.

Varying emphasis has been given to differing aspects of minimal cerebral dysfunction and amongst these have been the neurological, behavioural and educational factors. In a group of 85 children referred because of failure at school, including poor comprehension, reading and writing, there usually seemed to be adequate intelligence despite unsuccessful school learning (Boshes and Myklebust, 1964). Although parents often reported poor proficiency in learning to play and sometimes noted clumsiness and awkwardness, the findings included neurological integrity as revealed by clinical examination. Conners (1967) focused on diagnostic methods and principles of management and considered the frequently presumed evidence of prior central nervous system insult as a logical fallacy. The uses, limitations and pitfalls of psychodiagnostic tests incorporating scientific psychological jargon have been described by Mark (1969). Psychological and educational factors, particularly with regard to movement education, have been considered by Frostig (1971). Other aspects of interpretation of the problem with more peripheral considerations including its relationship to hydrocephalus and even neurohormonal function have been discussed by Pond (1961), Wigglesworth (1961), Hagberg (1962, 1963), Cizkova (1963), McFie (1963) and Paine and Oppé (1966).

Paine, Werry and Quay (1968) reported the study of 83 children with a diagnosis of minimal cerebral dysfunction. Minimal criteria for inclusion in this study were any one of the following:

1. Neurological signs
2. Abnormal EEG
3. Psychological findings of the type seen in organic encephalopathies plus either excessive clumsiness or an abnormal EEG.

There was a surprising lack of correlation between these data collected under different headings. The study suggested that the pattern of abnormalities observed in individual children reflected a complex matrix of underlying dimensions, some innate, some traumatic and some psychosocial. They warned that professionals should be circumspect in hypothesising about cerebral status in individual cases and concentrate on adequate psychosocial and educational assessment and rehabilitative programmes. An important conclusion was that the high degree of interrelatedness between abnormal history and neurological and EEG abnormalities as observed in children with major neurological abnormalities could not necessarily be extrapolated to children with minimal brain dysfunction.

The expression minimal cerebral dysfunction is an overall diagnostic term which highlights the fact that certain children, while not grossly impaired, exhibit limited deviations of intellect and behaviour of such a nature as to require special resources for their management and education. However, the existence of an underlying brain dysfunction in most instances is implied rather than proven. For this reason there are many—especially those involved in the education of children—who prefer to highlight the major problem and use the term 'learning disabilities' (Miller, 1969) rather than minimal cerebral dysfunction or the previous terminology, minimal brain damage.

Although minimal cerebral dysfunction might be a useful all-inclusive term, it is often inaccurately applied because, even though designated minimal, there is often a severe handicap to the child (Bax and MacKeith, 1963). The phrase also does not incorporate the concept of developmental failure. Hence the term 'neurodevelopmental dysfunction' may be used as a suitable alternative which could be applied collectively or singly to the various components such as developmental apraxia, developmental dysphasia, developmental dyscalculia and developmental dyslexia.

An excellent historical review of minimal cerebral dysfunction has been provided by Strother (1973). He observed the general agreement that children who have been included under the rubric of minimal brain dysfunction constitute a very heterogeneous group. It was suggested that the search for underlying common factors in pathology, aetiology, or response to treatment might be the next most important step, but that it might well depend on refinement of the concept of minimal brain dysfunction. It might be suggested here that conceptual refinement could begin by the more specific delineation of various syndromes within the total spectrum embracing this broad heterogenous group. In the epilogue to the monograph on minimal brain dysfunction, published by the New York Academy of Sciences, Masland (1973) lucidly summarised the present state of thought on the subject. He observed that a major emphasis of the conference had been on efforts to determine specific entities within this large nondescript group of individuals who have certain deviations of behaviour and methods of learning as their common characteristic. Clinicians should be alerted to the crucial need for neuropathological examination of individuals with minimal brain dysfunction who suffer accidental death because of the virtual absence of clinico-pathological correlations in this regard. Schain (1972) has made an attempt to sort out the semantic problems regarding diagnostic labels: "Recourse to arguments that the traditional neurological evaluation fails to detect 'subtle' disturbances of higher central nervous system functions is not an adequate substitute for providing solid evidence of neurological or neuropsychological abnormalities. If disturbed behaviour or learning is the phenomenon under consideration, it is best to categorise it under a term descriptive of the observed disorder such as learning disability or hyperactive behaviour syndrome". Wolff and Hurwitz (1973) suggested "that the functional significance of individual neurological signs and of combinations of such signs must be evaluated systematically in both normal children and children already identified as having social and academic difficulties, before any claims can be made for the validity of the minimal brain damage syndrome or any of its identifying features".

The broader concept of the classification of minimal cerebral dysfunction was discussed by Bakwin (1968a) who considered that the developmental disorders of maturity and language were manifestations of inborn errors in cerebral organisation. The lack of demonstrable anatomical lesions has never really been proven because of the dearth of pathological material for case studies, and it is true that any electroencephalographic changes noted in these cases may well have a physiological origin. It is assumed that the basis of developmental disorders is a delay or alteration in the maturation of those areas of the brain that govern motor co-ordination and language. Eventually it may be possible to relate myelination of the various areas of the brain to the assumption of their appropriate functions. The observed familial incidence is a further pointer towards a constitutional rather than a disruptive disturbance of function. The hypothesis is made that eventual recovery of normal function might be attributed to developmental delay, and incomplete improvement might be due to developmental abnormality. Denhoff (1971) classified the cerebral minimal syndromes (minimal brain dysfunction syndrome) as follows:

1. Hyperkinesis
2. Disorder of perception
3. Inefficient body awareness and control (leading to clumsiness)
4. Language dysfunctions
5. Emotional lability
6. Specific learning disabilities
7. Neurological abnormalities (presumably where recognisable or recognised neurological disease gives rise to 'soft signs' and electroencephalographic changes).

Against the background of the authoritative studies which have been quoted regarding the delineation and understanding of the term 'minimal cerebral dysfunction', an attempt will now be made to discuss more circumscribed abnormalities which may occur in individual children.

DISORDERS ALLIED TO DEVELOPMENTAL APRAXIA WITHIN THE SPECTRUM OF MINIMAL CEREBRAL DYSFUNCTION

Visuomotor Disability

The most comprehensive recent review on this subject has been made by Brenner and her co-authors in a series of papers (Brenner and Gillman, 1966, 1968; Brenner et al, 1967; Brenner, Gillman and Farrell, 1968). They recognised the existence of a condition in which children may suffer impairment of visuomotor function although no obvious neurological abnormality is diagnosed. The investigation was designed to provide normative data on the range of visuomotor abilities of a large sample of schoolchildren and to obtain a test battery to select subjects with specific disabilities in visuomotor performance from a normal school population. In a representative diverse sample of 810 eight-year-old children attending the Cambridgeshire area of England, 77 children fell into a group whose performance on the test battery was considerably worse than would have been expected from their IQ scores. It was suggested that pupils with a good verbal ability and very poor visuomotor performance were likely to be as severely handicapped as children with the opposite imbalance of skills. It appears that at the age of 11 years a combination of good verbal intelligence with poor visuomotor ability results in poor or indifferent scholastic achievement. Both verbal and perceptual motor abilities are necessary for academic success at 10 to 11 years of age. Children in the lower six or seven per cent of visuomotor ability were found to be significantly inferior with regard to spatial judgement and manual skills and to present a variety of educational problems especially with regard to spelling, writing and arithmetic, although reading was as a rule adequate. Other adjectives used to describe these children included clumsy, untidy, careless, slovenly, awkward, inept, irritating, difficult, unpopular and lacking in self confidence. The disparity between various motor abilities is exemplified by the description of one child who was very dexterous with tweezers but quite unable to juxtapose forefinger and thumb out of context. Further examples of apraxia included one child slow in imitating hand positions and another at facial grimaces. Abercrombie (1964) discussed visuomotor disability within the setting of spastic cerebral palsy where evidence suggested that a spastic disorder was likely to lead to a greater than average difficulty with visuomotor tasks.

Developmental Gerstmann's Syndrome

Gerstmann (1924, 1927, 1940) described the syndrome of finger agnosia, disorientation for right and left, agraphia and acalculia for which there was ample anatomical neuropathological correlation implying disruption of the dominant angular gyrus. Spillane (1942) described the case of congenital Gerstmann's syndrome in a man who had slow early development. One cannot extrapolate from the anatomical localisation in patients with acquired Gerstmann's syndrome to patients with the developmental syndrome where the disturbance more likely is in neurophysiological organisation. Critchley (1953) also described a congenital variety of Gerstmann's syndrome un-accompanied by any other neurological abnormality.

Kinsbourne (1968) propounded the concept of developmental Gerstmann's syndrome with varying manifestations of Gerstmann's tetrad. He stated that many of the children were 'clumsy' without showing identifiable neurological deficits such as ataxia or spasticity. Kinsbourne and Warrington (1963a, b) referred to children of normal intelligence without gross physical handicap who failed to learn to read or write at the expected age because of a deficiency in one or more of their physiological functions that contributed to the acquisition of reading and writing skill. Although the functional deficits found in the children were thought to be remarkably like those of adult patients with acquired Gertsmann's syndrome, it was conceded that the syndrome did not have the same anatomical implications in childhood as in the adult setting. The highest incidence of failure with tests of finger agnosia were in children where there was a probable neurological basis to their reading retardation and the lowest incidence was in those with deprived backgrounds of emotional instability. The authors had shown previously that finger agnosia was due to an inability to identify the fingers on the basis of their relative positions in sequence on the hand.

Benton (1959) commented on the frequency of developmental disorders of right–left discrimination and finger localisation. Defects in finger localisation may be associated with an apraxia of finger movement. Benton frequently noted indexterity in patients with difficulty in right–left discrimination and devised a 32-item test with five components to test right–left orientation.

Albitreccia (1958, 1959) has been more concerned with congenital disorders of the body image which clinically bear some relationship to the concept of developmental Gerstmann's syndrome.

Developmental Dyscalculia

This condition pertains to children with the isolated phenomenon of impaired mathematical ability. They do not appear to be referred for neurological study, presumably because the disorder is more socially acceptable in contrast to the problems of impaired ability to read, write or spell. The definitive writings on this subject are by Cohn (1961a, b, 1964, 1968) who has found various forms of apraxia and dysarthria in the afflicted subjects. In acquired dyscalculia, the condition may result from the lesions in widely disparate regions of the brain, including those disturbing the physiological control of the visual apparatus where there is a profound alteration of the processes of arithmetic 'order'. Memory processes are also important in the concept of eucalculia. The differential characteristic of children with developmental dyscalculia is a prolongation of the time and increase in the amount of energy required to achieve an adequate use of numbers. Among the several manifestations, Cohn has described malformed or large number symbols, strephosymbolia, and inability to sum single integers. The changes are basically similar to the elementary disturbances Cohn has also described in *acquired* dyscalculia, namely: (1) failure to develop the ability to recognise number symbols, usually as part of a general language dissolution; (2) failure to remember the basic operations, or the use of operator and separator symbols; (3) the inability to recall tables and to 'carry' numbers in multiplication; and (4) the inability to maintain number sequence in calculation. In remediation of this condition it has been advocated that we should teach according to the child's strengths as opposed to his weaknesses, and improve it with proponents.

Developmental Dyslexia

The original occurrence of dyslexia must date from antiquity when humans first learned to communicate through written symbols. Morgan (1896) described 'congenital word blindness' in an intelligent boy aged 14 years who apparently had an isolated dyslexia comprising inability to read simple words or write to dictation unassociated with ocular or visual defect or dyscalculia.

Although some authors regard developmental dyslexia as a distinct entity which should not be considered within the category of minimal cerebral dysfunction, evidence has accrued to the contrary. Kawi and Pasamanick (1958) have shown that many of the abnormalities of pregnancy, labour and delivery which are thought to be important in stillbirth, neonatal death and cerebral palsy are also present in a number of neuropsychiatric disorders. They found that 16.6 per cent of a series of 205 children with reading retardation had complications during the mother's pregnancy such as pre-eclampsia, bleeding or hypertension. As a control group of normal readers showed an incidence of 1.5 per cent, it was deduced that there was a relatively benign form of brain damage leading to faulty speech and congenital dyslexia. Amongst three groups of poor readers isolated by Rabinovich et al (1954) were those with 'secondary reading retardation' due to 'brain damage'. Ingram

(1960) maintained that reading and writing difficulties encountered in children with cerebral palsy were similar in type to those observed in normal children, but with a tendency to increased frequency, severity and recalcitrance. Goldberg, Marshall and Sims (1960) have discussed the role of 'brain damage' in congenital dyslexia.

Hansen (1963) carried out a preliminary study of 55 pupils in a school for physically handicapped children, all 10 years of age or more and with IQs exceeding 80. The subjects had a high incidence of reading difficulty, dyscalculia, right–left confusion, finger agnosia and constructional apraxia, suggesting that parietal lobe dysfunction was encountered more frequently than in children with specific dyslexia (developmental dyslexia). This author also estimated that about 10 per cent of all pupils in ordinary schools needed special remedial reading classes. Hallgren (1950) had previously worked on the hypothesis that the incidence of specific dyslexia in the normal population was 10 per cent. Gooddy and Reinhold (1961) had emphasised right–left disorientation of varying degree in children with congenital (developmental) dyslexia.

McFie (1952) in using the Phi test of lateral dominance in visual function, described by Jasper and Raney (1937), found close correlation between hemispheric dominance as indicated by the test and by the subject's handedness. The results suggested that in dyslexics the neurophysiological organisation corresponding to dominance has not been established normally in either hemisphere.

Critchley (1967, 1968a, b, c, 1970) provided masterly reviews on the role of organic brain disease in the aetiology of developmental dyslexia. He felt that most neurologists would be reluctant to visualise in developmental dyslexia any focal brain lesion, dysplastic, traumatic or otherwise, despite the analogy of the acquired cases of alexia after cerebral damage. To do so would be to ignore the important factor of immaturity as applied to chronological age, cortical development and processes of learning. On the other hand he recognised that inordinate clumsiness did occur (34 of 125 cases of his personal series). Against the acceptance of an hypothesis of 'minimal' brain damage he forwarded the following arguments:

1. No history of perinatal problems or of post-natal trauma or disease might be forthcoming
2. Positive family history
3. Soft neurologic signs were often not demonstrable
4. EEG abnormalities were inconstant, mild and probably not significant.

The contention that congenital dyslexia does not arise from an acquired pathological lesion of the brain has been supported further by the observations of Hermann (1956), Hermann and Norrie (1958), Gutelius and Layman (1960) and Kerr (1897). Bender (1958) discussed a wider neuropsychological concept of developmental dyslexia. She alluded to the many controversies as to whether the basic cause was related to the method of teaching, personality problems or ego defects or maturational lag, and found them awkward in their motor control or motility, thereby supporting earlier observations by De Hirsch (1954).

The lack of clinicopathological correlation in this syndrome will probably lead to much conjecture on aetiology for many years to come. Even our present methods of neuropathological assessment may not yield information which might only be forthcoming after the development of more refined techniques of analysis.

Originally the concept of developmental dyslexia was reasonably well circumscribed, referring to children with an isolated difficulty in reading and writing when other parameters of neurological function were intact. Furthermore, children with primary visual, behavioural, orthopaedic and other sundry disturbances which might contribute to the problems of reading and writing were excluded from consideration within this group. With the burgeoning enthusiasm towards the recognition and treatment of children with learning difficulties akin to developmental dyslexia and even mental retardation, the popular concept of 'dyslexia' was expanded. In the attempt to achieve greater social acceptance for individual children with a wide variety of learning disorders, they have been labelled inappropriately as 'dyslexics', with a consequent blurring of the borders of this hitherto specifically defined entity. The euphemism 'dyslexia', similar to the term autism, has become a term of disparagement, after its popular usage extended to implications of mental deficiency. Because of the misusage of the term dyslexia it has been relegated unfortunately by some educationists and psychologists to the scrap-heap of undesirable terminologies. This attitude has pervaded into the general population, so that the child with specific developmental dyslexia is included with the paradoxically less specific group of Specific Learning Disabilities. While there is every justification in redesignating dyslexia associations and specific learning disability groups with wider terms of reference, there is no justification in dispensing with the specificity of the term dyslexia in identifying many individuals within the broader group.

Developmental Speech Dysfunction

Orton (1937) mentioned motor speech delay and stuttering as two of the six commonly occurring developmental disorders. The other frequently associated problems that he described comprised reading disability, writing disability, word deafness and abnormal clumsiness or developmental apraxia. Morely et al (1955) reviewed 278 cases of delay in speaking in childhood and classified them under the following main headings: (1) disorders arising from deafness; (2) aphasia; (3) dysarthria; (4) dyslalia; and (5) stammering. In patients with developmental aphasia there was a high incidence of birth injury, defective articulation and delayed and defective speech in the family. The condition is characterised by gross delay in the acquisition of speech in both its receptive and expressive components. The social isolation of these children because of their inability to communicate except perhaps through written symbols may be associated with extreme frustration. With behavioural anomalies characterised by increasing dependence and yet social withdrawal, the condition of autism might at first be suspected.

Slow and clumsy articulation arising from dysfunction of the muscles used in speech is characteristic of dysarthria. Morley (1957) further classified disorders of articulation into: (1) developmental dysarthria; (2) developmental articulatory apraxia; (3) dyslalia; (4) defective articulation due to deficient hearing; and (5) defective articulation due to various structural abnormalities. In essence the distinction between the first and second of these latter categories is that developmental articulatory apraxia is due to a disturbance higher on the effector side of motor speech function and may be associated with apraxia as opposed to weakness, spasticity or inco-ordination of the tongue, lips and palate.

Morley, Court and Miller (1954) studied 18 children with isolated dysarthria. They found that a familial tendency was common whereas birth injury, prematurity and emotional disturbances were not significant in aetiology. Twelve of the 18 children exhibited abnormal movements of the lips, tongue and palate and in the remaining six children, these articulatory muscles were normal on voluntary movements carried out on request, but clumsy and awkward when the children attempted more complex and rapid movements of articulation. Some of the children had associated disorders of language including dyslexia. There was a tendency to gradual improvement especially with the more intelligent subjects.

Among the theories regarding the origin of stammering, Andrews and Harris (1964) considered the possibility of minimal cerebral dysfunction in which minor perceptual abnormality may be contributory. Alternative aetiological theories which were propounded included psychoneurotic conflict and maladaptive learning. Although with stammerers there is fundamentally no disturbance of the central formulation of speech or its articulation, stammering may be a presenting feature of acquired dysphasic and dysarthric conditions.

Ingram (1968) applied the term 'developmental speech disorder syndrome' to children from a normal environment who, despite normal health and average or superior intelligence, were slow to acquire speech. He believed that most clinicians would consider a child to have retarded speech development if there were no words by the age of two years and no phrases by three years. Many of the patients were observed to manifest 'soft' neurological signs.

The Choreiform Syndrome

Prechtl and Stemmer (1962) had described an identifiable neurological syndrome in 50 children with habitual clumsiness and choreiform movements. They had hyperkinetic behaviour and poor educational performance with specific difficulties in learning to read and write.

Developmental Hyperactivity

Werry (1968) defined this syndrome as a total daily motor activity which was significantly greater than the norm. Anderson (1963) found minor neurological abnormalities in a high proportion of hyperkinetic patients and postulated that the entire syndrome was due to a lack of adequate integration of various types of perceptual modalities resulting from minimal brain damage. Ounsted (1955) has made reference to the high proportion of patients with this type of overactive behaviour, but without gross neurological signs, where lesions in one or the other temporal lobe could be demonstrated by electro-encephalography or by operation. Overactive behaviour has now itself become an indication of possible or even probable 'brain damage' (Ingram, 1956; Bradley, 1957; Bingley, 1958; Falconer and Cavanagh, 1959). Bakwin (1967) included developmental hyperactivity among the developmental disorders which are inborn delays in the organisation of cerebral function. Clumsiness in these children may be due to haste, impatience, low frustration levels and also restlessness.

THE CLUMSY CHILD SYNDROME WITHIN THE SPECTRUM OF CEREBRAL PALSY

As neurological signs manifest in many children categorised within the 'clumsy child syndrome', the syndrome itself could be regarded as part of the spectrum of cerebral palsy which usually refers to the more overt manifestations of a congenital motor disorder. Walton, Ellis and Court (1962) and Dare and Gordon (1970) have discussed this concept. It has been recognised for many years that children with cerebral palsy often exhibit agnosic and apraxic defects which compound the problem of integration of movement (Lord, 1937; Strauss and Werner, 1942; Strauss and Lehtinen, 1947; Dunsdon, 1952; Cruikshank et al, 1957; Woods, 1957; Crothers and Paine, 1959; Daryn, 1961).

Just as abnormal clumsiness might be regarded as a possible manifestation of minimal cerebral dysfunction, the latter in turn might qualify as a forme fruste of cerebral palsy. Without pathological confirmation, this notion can only remain conjectural and in any case it does not encompass the possibility that a defect of maturation of neurophysiological organisation must be the basic underlying aetiology in some cases of minimal cerebral dysfunction (Knobloch and Pasamanick, 1959; Clements, 1966b; Paine and Oppé, 1966). Other partial syndromes of minimal cerebral dysfunction akin to developmental apraxia often yield more substantive evidence of underlying focal or diffuse encephalopathy. Thus, perceptual disorders have been discussed within this context by Bortner and Birch (1960, 1962), Skatvedt (1960), Wedell (1961), Williams (1961) and Abercrombie (1964). Bingley (1958) and Anderson (1963) have referred to a neuropathological basis for hyperkinesia.

SPECIFIC LEARNING DISABILITY

Although the two terms are not synonymous, the educationist's counterpart of the concept of minimal cerebral dysfunction is specific learning disability.

The latter refers to the educational problems which may be encountered by the child with minimal cerebral dysfunction. These children are increasingly referred to physicians mainly to identify whether physical factors are contributing to failure in school performance. In many cases it is the prerogative of the paediatrician or the neurologist to collect all the available multidisciplinary information from school teachers, psychologists and therapists in order to achieve diagnosis. From the practical viewpoint, in most cases of learning disorder, the medical clinician makes his main contribution in the field of diagnosis rather than management. Of special importance is his ability to reassure both parent and child that there is no serious or progressive underlying physical disorder. The problems of further management are nearly always referred back to the educationist. Occasionally the medical practitioner may contribute significantly by supervising the administration of drugs and ensuring the correction of other chronic physical disabilities especially related to vision and hearing. That is not to say that the neurological consultant should shirk his role as an expert advisor on theories relating to neurological dysfunction in learning problems of children. There is substantial evidence that neurological, educational and environmental factors significantly contribute to the problem of poor learning performance in large numbers of children with normal mental abilities (Schain, 1972).

CHAPTER TWO

Developmental Clumsiness

HISTORY AND DESCRIPTIONS

The concept of developmental clumsiness has been documented since at least the earlier part of this century when Collier (see Ford, 1966) used the term 'congenital maladroitness'. With regard to isolated developmental neurological disturbances in general, perhaps one of the earliest descriptions is incorporated in Morgan's (1896) description of 'a case of congenital word blindness'. Kramer and Pollnow (1932) were amongst the original writers on the subject of minimal cerebral dysfunction. Following the pioneer work of Lord (1937), recognition of the perceptual, educational and personality difficulties of patients suffering from cerebral palsy attracted great interest. It was demonstrated that some patients could be shown to have such difficulties as a result of 'brain damage' without manifest abnormalities on neurological examination. Other authors have appreciated that perceptual disorders are common in children with cerebral palsy (Strauss and Lehtinen, 1947; Dunsdon, 1952; Cruikshank et al, 1957; Woods, 1957).

Orton (1937) recognised that disorders of praxis and gnosis resulted in clumsiness of physical performance and that this clumsiness was clearly distinct from that arising from pyramidal, extrapyramidal or cerebellar dysfunction. He considered that 'abnormal clumsiness' or developmental apraxia was one of the six commonly occurring developmental disorders. The other frequently associated disorders that he recognised were in the general sphere of communication. Williams (1961) expanded on the theme of perceptual disorders in children with hemiplegia and made particular mention of visuoperceptual disability in these subjects. Hagberg's observations (1962, 1963) on hydrocephalic children in relation to children with recognised cerebral palsy who have agnosic and apraxic defects are also relevant in this context.

Annell (1949) described a child who played truant on days coinciding with class gymnastics because he felt incapable of dressing and undressing and taking a shower after the lesson. This author described motor dysfunctions

35

occurring in children with otherwise good intelligence. These dysfunctions produced difficulties at school and prevented normal play and association with other children. They were interpreted as symptoms of either organic immaturity or of cerebral lesions. She felt that the deviation from the normal motor development of the child indicated the presence of organic exciting factors. Eight per cent of 600 patients between the ages of 6 and 17 years in an outpatient department of child psychiatry manifested motor dysfunction. This did not include gross organic lesions which had given rise to paralysis, spasticity, or poor motor development related to mental retardation. In subdividing the cases of motor dysfunction, she used the term 'motor infantilism'. There were altogether seven other rather artificial and arbitrary subgroups.

Doll (1951) had probably observed apraxic children when he described the syndrome of neuromuscular impairment other than typical cerebral palsy which was not easy to recognise. He remarked that these defects sometimes could be accompanied by others in the field of receptive experience leading to visual, auditory and language handicaps, and thought that a confusion of cerebral laterality might be responsible for the condition. Benton (1959) had noticed that lack of dexterity was frequent in patients with difficulty in right—left discrimination. Albitreccia (1958, 1959) provided a very positive method of approach to helping these children with therapeutic exercises to overcome disturbances of body image.

Walton (1961, 1963) was one of the first to designate the syndrome by the term 'clumsy children'. It was the report given by Walton, Ellis and Court (1962) on a group of such cases which provided the original impetus and inspiration for the work of this book. Their case reports of 'clumsy children' who have been categorised as afflicted with developmental apraxia and agnosia were supplemented later by Gubbay et al (1965). Illingworth (1963, 1968), Reuben and Bakwin (1968), Bakwin (1968a) and Dare and Gordon (1970) have all defined the syndrome as a precise entity whereas Paine (1968) would have regarded developmental clumsiness as one of the syndromes within the ambit of 'minimal cerebral damage'. A succinct review was featured in the *British Medical Journal* (1962) in which it was stressed that clumsy children were not at all uncommon.

As part of the wider concept of 'central processing dysfunction' in children, the U.S. Department of Health, Education and Welfare has alluded to the problems of clumsiness resulting from disturbances of visual processing and 'haptic' processing, the latter referring to the integration of cutaneous and kinaesthetic information. A very real attempt has been made to define the problems of 'minimal brain dysfunction in children' (Clements, 1966a) when broader concepts of developmental clumsiness are considered.

Berko (1966) considered that apraxia could be disruptive to both central organisation and discriminative learning. A group of 85 children referred because of school failure, but usually with adequate intelligence, were often reported by their parents as clumsy, awkward and showing poor proficiency in learning to play (Boshes and Myklebust, 1964).

Interest was focused on the problem of the clumsy child in a monograph on minimal cerebral dysfunction (Bax and MacKeith, 1963). Illingworth (1963) appreciated that clumsiness was one of the handicaps which might pass unrecognised by the schoolteacher and that the affected child was apt to get into serious trouble. Ingram (1963) made a very sound critical review on 'chronic brain syndromes in childhood other than cerebral palsy, epilepsy and mental defect'. In his provisional classification of such chronic brain syndromes, he included specific clumsiness, as well as specific developmental dyslexia and specific speech retardation under the heading of 'defined clinical syndromes with *inconstant* evidence of brain abnormality'. Köng (1963) mentioned that in very many school classes there would be found a clumsy child, who lacked concentration, had slow reactions, substandard handwriting, poor performance and awkward movements in gymnastics. Wigglesworth (1963) stressed the importance of diagnosis because the afflicted children found great difficulty in coping with their environmental circumstances and it was also difficult for their parents and teachers to cope. He maintained that often a simple explanation of the clinical diagnosis and the symptoms, perhaps with a demonstration of minimal signs, gave back to the child a feeling of self-respect.

Brenner and Gillman (1966) have carried out surveys of visuomotor disability in schoolchildren where clumsiness has been a very important presenting abnormality. In fact the characteristic most frequently remarked upon in these children was clumsiness either in gait or movement or in fine motor control or both. A large proportion were noted for untidiness and careless or slovenly work (see also Brenner et al, 1967; Brenner, Gillman and Farrell, 1968). Rutter, Tizard and Whitmore (1970) in their epidemiological surveys remarked that clumsiness may occur in isolation in children without cerebral palsy and of normal intelligence.

In a further follow-up control study on 14 children (Brenner, Gillman and Farrell, 1968) clumsiness or poor motor co-ordination was found in a high proportion of the children, but was virtually absent in the controls. These authors supported the contention by Gubbay et al (1965) that developmental agnosic and apraxic syndromes were much commoner than was generally supposed. Frostig (1963) emphasised the manifestation of clumsiness in children with disturbances of visual perception. Perceptual motor impairment was the second most common of 10 characteristics cited by various authors within the definition of the minimal brain dysfunction syndrome (Clements, 1966a). Zangwill (1960a) described a girl who was clumsy, but medical opinion was that the disorder was psychological and did not warrant further action. She had very little neurological disorder in generally accepted terms, but psychological testing revealed that her clumsiness was linked with a very profound visuospatial disorder.

Kirk (1968) probably would have included specific clumsiness within his concept of 'learning disability' which he defined as a specific retardation or disorder in one or more of the processes of speech, language, perception, behaviour, reading, spelling, writing or arithmetic. Bakwin (1968a) observed that children with developmental clumsiness were unhappy because their school grades suffered owing to poor handwriting and because of ineptness in sports. He stressed the importance of early recognition and considered that better parent–child relations would arise from giving the parents of afflicted children some understanding of the nature of developmental disorders. In describing the more specific disturbance of 'developmental Gerstmann syndrome', Kinsbourne (1968) revealed that many of the children affected were 'clumsy' without showing identifiable neurological deficits such as ataxia or spasticity.

Paine (1968) has been one of the chief workers in the field of minimal cerebral dysfunction. He remarked that conventional neurological examination usually showed no abnormality of the standard signs such as in the cranial nerves and reflexes, although a certain number of patients had extensor plantar responses or hyperreflexia. General clumsiness was frequently noted and was likely to be more conspicuous for fine muscle co-ordination than for gross functions such as running, jumping and hopping. Writing, drawing, catching a ball, tying laces, doing up buttons might all be affected. Paine and Oppé (1966) observed that mentally retarded children were generally clumsier than children of normal intelligence, although some were quite agile.

Masland (1969a) referred to the significant qualitative differences in the abilities of children, which have been slow in receiving adequate recognition. Clumsy children would probably qualify for his statement that "with special instruction, appropriate to the specific characteristics of the individual child, many are able to surmount those difficulties and move ahead to normal or superior academic and social achievement".

Paine and Oppé (1966) and Critchley (1967, 1968a, b) have cogently drawn attention to the imprecision of the term 'clumsiness' to a neurologist and the difficulty in the evaluation of this symptom. Critchley (1970) described a general gaucherie or awkwardness among the motility disorders which may beset dyslexic children. The gait may be shambling, the child may run in an ungainly fashion and frequently tumble. Manual dexterity may be so maladroit as to raise the suspicion of a 'congenital' type of motor dyspraxia, but on the other hand inordinate clumsiness was described as 'anything but an invariable symptom'. Klasen (1972) also referred to generalised awkwardness in some children with specific dyslexia. Greater precision in a neurological sense was shown by European writers on the subject of developmental apraxia (Wallon and Denjean, 1958; Bergès, 1966; Di Cagno and Ravetto, 1967; Stambak et al, 1964).

Certain features of the syndrome of developmental clumsiness have been emphasised. Amongst these are the almost consistently higher verbal than performance scores in the Wechsler Intelligence Scale for Children (Walton, Ellis and Court, 1962; Reuben and Bakwin, 1968; Paine, 1968; Brenner, Gillman and Farrell, 1968; Dare and Gordon, 1970). A relative disparity between clumsiness for one physical act and dexterity for another has been observed by Brenner, Gillman and Farrell (1968). A paucity or even a complete lack of signs elicited from routine conventional neurological examination is an important negative feature of this syndrome (Lord, 1937; Drew, 1956; Zangwill, 1960a; Kennard, 1960; Köng, 1963; Ingram, 1963; Boshes and Myklebust, 1964; Lucas, Rodin and Simson, 1965; Clements, 1966a; Bakwin, 1968a; Coppele and Isom, 1968; Mac Keith, 1968; Paine, 1968; Paine, Werry and Quay, 1968). It might be mentioned in passing that conversely Gubbay, Lobascher and Kingerlee (1970a, b) in a neurological appraisal of autistic children had found a moderate incidence of relatively subtle neurological signs, whereas autism does not ordinarily have the connotation of a neurological disorder.

Mild choreiform movements, which could be regarded as an accentuation of the physiological chorea of normal children, have been observed by Brenner, Gillman and Farrell (1968) and Dare and Gordon (1970). These choreiform movements have been considered in differing contexts, as with hyperactive behaviour and learning difficulties by Timme (1948), Prechtl and Stemmer (1962) and Stemmer (1964). The significance of these movements has been questioned by Rutter, Graham and Birch (1966), Rutter, Tizard and Whitmore (1970) and Wolff and Hurwitz (1966). The assessment of mild chorea in children is always difficult because it is subjective and the paediatric neurologist recognises the gradually diminishing tendency to physiological chorea with increasing age. A degree of choreiform movement is nearly always evident in a child below the age of eight years and it certainly can be a variable manifestation in any one child depending upon extraneous factors, e.g. emotion as with physiological tremor.

That the syndrome of developmental clumsiness has acquired recognition is evidenced by its acceptance in standard modern neurological textbooks (Ford, 1966; Walton, 1966; Brain and Walton, 1969; Elliot, 1971) which allude to its relationships within the spectrum of minimal cerebral dysfunction. Ford (1966) discussed this entity under the term 'congenital maladroitness', whereas Walton has preferred the term 'developmental apraxia and agnosia'. In the United States there is even State and Federal legislation specifically relating to the field of 'Specific Learning Disabilities' (Kass, Hall and Simches, 1969) which would certainly encompass the problem of developmental apraxia and agnosia.

Thus, many influential authorities in the field of developmental neurology have been fully cognisant of the challenge of the 'clumsy child'. Although some have accepted a broader concept of developmental cerebral dysfunction within which clumsiness might manifest as a dominant characteristic, the syndrome often has been considered as a specific entity. In fact there are distinct advantages in delineating developmental clumsiness from all other forms of developmental cerebral dysfunction, for the problems of these children are more specific and require special considerations in management. Although other associated disabilities such as speech, behavioural and learning problems frequently coexist, there is a very definite central theme in this condition, as for example in developmental dyslexia.

DEFINITIONS

In the context of this report, the 'clumsy child' is to be regarded as one who is mentally normal, without bodily deformity, and whose physical strength, sensation, and co-ordination are virtually normal by the standards of routine conventional neurological assessment, but whose ability to perform skilled, purposive movement is impaired. This type of clumsiness is designated by the neurological term apraxia. As praxis and gnosis are so closely allied and are interdependent in the performance of skilled movement a defect in one will result in disturbance of the other, either because of impairment of integration or kinaesthetic feedback. Both terms 'apraxia' and 'agnosia' can be applied to the manifest disabilities of these children. The term 'developmental' implies a congenital or early acquired defect or disorder in the development of a particular function. The functions in this context refer to gnosis and praxis and hence the terminology 'developmental apraxia and agnosia' can be justified as the precise nosology pertaining to the clumsiness of these children, or more succinctly 'developmental apraxic ataxia'.

The terms apraxia and agnosia in adult neurology imply the loss of a once intact function, whereas in developmental neurological jargon it is implied that these functions have never developed normally. Russell (1960) maintained that the term apraxia was used more satisfactorily to describe the loss of a previously acquired skill and certainly should be distinguished clearly from the inability to develop motor skills in cases of brain defect. Thus, there could be valid objection to the term 'developmental apraxia and agnosia', but it is expedient to employ established jargon in order to avoid further confusion which could arise from coining a new term. Furthermore, there is a closely parallel precedent in the usage of terms such as developmental dyslexia and developmental dyscalculia. The word 'clumsy' does not have sufficient precision to be acceptable as a scientific neurological term, because clumsiness may be the end result of a large number of differing neurological defects. However, it can be a most useful expression in conveying the message to parents and teachers alike, provided its lack of specificity is fully appreciated. 'Ataxia', meaning unsteadiness or unco-ordinated movement, is often equated with cerebellar abnormalities. However, the terms 'sensory ataxia' and 'spastic ataxia' are quite as acceptable in neurological parlance as 'cerebellar ataxia'. There should be thus no objection to the terms 'apraxic' and/or 'agnosic ataxia' because apraxia and agnosia may also give rise to comparable derangement of volitional movement amounting to clumsiness.

As there is a very broad spectrum of motor ability or dexterity in the juvenile population, it is difficult to determine the arbitrary point in the scale below which a child might be regarded as significantly clumsy. The same problem exists with all biological functions which have a spread of normal variation. A composite function such as motor performance is even more difficult to assess in absolute terms because there can be no single parameter and only artificial arbitrary standards can be instituted. Ultimately it can only be a matter of opinion as to whether a particular child's clumsiness is a problem, for it depends upon the relative standards of his environment as well as its competitiveness. A particular child's indexterity only becomes a problem when it results in failure to satisfy his particular environmental requirements. Nevertheless, arbitrary standards of motor performance are necessary for the broad assessment of individual children or for screening large groups of children such as entire school populations.

Arising from these considerations are two important corollaries which form the basis of much of the material in this book. Firstly, we ought to know the magnitude and prevalence of the problem of developmental clumsiness; and secondly, we ought to be able to employ simple screening tests which would facilitate the recognition of these children. Although several standardised tests of motor ability have been developed previously or are still in the process of development, there remains a definite need for simple tests which can be administered rapidly by any responsible person of professional status. These tests would have to be suitable for employment by a medical practitioner as a brief, uncomplicated consulting room procedure, or by a school medical officer or physical education teacher for screening large numbers of children.

Apraxia and Agnosia

The performance of skilled or complicated acts—those which require higher cerebral control in either the motor or sensory spheres, together with psychic elaboration of the ideational plan—is considered as an eupractic function. The perfect execution of such acts is known as eupraxia; a disturbance of the execution of skilled acts is apraxia (DeJong, 1967). Apraxia ('mind blindness') may be defined as the inability to move a certain part of the body in accordance with the proposed purpose, the motility of the part being otherwise preserved.

Ellis (1967) defined apraxia as the inability to carry out a willed, voluntary movement despite intact sensory and motor pathways concerned in the control of the movement and the individual understanding what is intended. Movements therefore are clumsy and the individual is slow to learn skilled movements. Wernicke (1874) propounded that complex activities were learned by means of connections between a small number of functional regions which dealt with the primary motor and sensory activities. Denny-Brown (1966) asserted that the defect of apraxia was not in the organisation of movement, but in the ability to translate a proposition into action. The propositional nature of the task was thus at fault and the patient had other difficulties in comprehending the nature of propositional requests, demonstrating that the defect is primarily related to perception or agnosia. The individual also had no difficulty in performing spontaneous tasks. Barsch (1967) considered that the concept of inability to motor-plan was covered by the term apraxia. Heilman (1973) suggested that what may be at fault in ideational apraxia is the process or processes which occur between language comprehension and motor encoding.

Agnosias of all types are characterised by the loss of ability to comprehend the meaning or recognise the importance of various types of stimulation, and are actually perceptive defects. Gnosis is the higher synthesis of sensory impulses, with resulting appreciation and perception of stimuli. Ellis (1967) defined agnosia simply as an inability to recognise the significance of sensory stimuli. Because agnosias interfere with sensory perception, they also interfere with motor performance and may cause not only delayed motor development but also clumsiness of movement.

The term apraxia has really been 'borrowed' from adult neurology and, as already mentioned, Russell (1960) suggested that it could be used to describe more satisfactorily the loss of a previously acquired skill and should certainly be clearly distinguished from the inability to develop motor skills. Zangwill

(1960a) gave further support to Russell in calling attention to the dangers of making too close an identification between disorders of development or maturation on the one hand and true dissolution, i.e. the breakdown of established skills in older children or adults, on the other. The term 'developmental' therefore should always be used to qualify the neurological defect which most closely resembles the acquired disorder, e.g. developmental apraxia, developmental aphasia, developmental alexia.

Walton (1963) felt that it was never possible to distinguish apraxia from agnosia completely, for defects of recognition almost invariably resulted in defects of execution, and Brain (1961) has aptly employed the term 'apractognosia'. Kephart (1971) also subscribed to the view that perceptual skills and motor skills should not be considered as two separate activities since perceptual skills provided continual feedback for co-ordinating motor movements.

The anatomical and physiological explanations of apraxia are varied. A lesion of the posterior divisions of the sensorimotor region (area 4) results in disturbances of spatial integration or of kinaesthetic schemes of movement upon which motor behaviour is based. Motor impulses lose selectivity and are conducted to agonists and antagonists simultaneously (Denny-Brown, 1958). Schiller (1969), in a discussion on apraxia, propounded that simple clumsiness was associated with disturbances of the pre-central and post-central areas for the contralateral hand and/or foot. Nielsen (1962) and Langworthy (1970) assumed that a quite different pathogenesis was the basis of the production of developmental apraxia in contradistinction to acquired apraxia in that there could well be a physiological rather than an anatomical basis for the symptomatology.

Whereas Geschwind (1965) hypothesised that many disorders of the higher functions of the nervous system, such as the aphasias, apraxias and agnosias, might be studied most productively as disturbances produced by anatomical disconnection of primary receptive and motor areas from one another, the developmental apraxias might well imply that these connections have never actually been established. Lissauer (1889) divided the agnosias into aperceptive and associative, or disorders of primary and secondary recognition; and Geschwind's thesis would favour the view that agnosias are indeed associative disorders.

Classification

The term 'clumsy children' could be expressed more aptly as 'abnormally clumsy children'. Abnormal clumsiness in children occurs for a large variety of reasons, but may be isolated and apparently constitutional. It should be regarded as an all-inclusive end-product of differing aetiologies implying heterogeneous aetiology and as an inconstant manifestation of 'minimal cerebral dysfunction'.

Bax and MacKeith (1963) and Ingram (1963) have alluded to the challenge of the problematical multiplicity of classification concepts (Stevens and Birch,

1957; Abrams, 1968) which also was referred to more recently by Block (1971). Gomez (1967) whimsically entitled his article 'Minimal Cerebral Dysfunction (Maximal Neurologic Confusion)' and aptly drew attention to the four dimensions of the definition of a disorder: aetiological, anatomical, pathophysiological and functional. He encouraged specific descriptions of a patient's various disabilities.

ABNORMAL CLUMSINESS IN CHILDHOOD

In more severely afflicted children there may be a history of perinatal abnormalities including toxaemia of pregnancy, dysmaturity, prolonged labour and abnormal delivery. In milder cases perinatal difficulties of these types are more likely to occur fortuitously as is a history of childhood cerebral disorders including head injury, meningitis, encephalitis or epilepsy. More often than by chance, there may be a family history of clumsiness or related developmental dysfunction. Of the 56 clumsy children described in Chapter 4, there were three in a sibship of six children who were included in the study.

There is often slowness in the acquisition of developmental motor milestones, but usually the delay is only mild. Speech also tends to develop tardily and at first indistinctly, especially if there is an associated developmental dysarthria. Except in extreme cases the condition may be inapparent in the first three or four years of life. The frequent falls after first learning to walk and the tendency to bump into objects and strike the head repeatedly on tables and doors is usually initially dismissed by parents, who regard the situation as a variation of normal rather than a special idiosyncrasy. Perhaps greater anxiety may accrue when it is observed that the child is unable to manipulate door handles and door knobs with normal facility.

In the kindergarten and pre-school age groups, the clumsy child first becomes seriously challenged by the performance of physical tasks to which he is unequal. The more tenacious and persistent of these children eventually succeed. Unfortunately the timid or temperamental young child becomes readily frustrated from constant failure and may become diffident in performing manual tasks. Alternatively the sense of frustration may be severe enough to produce emotional outbursts such as temper tantrums or aggravate an already underlying tendency to hyperactivity.

The problems reach their zenith in the earlier school years. The child is increasingly expected to look after his own personal needs at home as well as to cope with the demands of motor skills both within the classroom and on the playground. His mother at first may deride him repeatedly for ineffectual tooth brushing and hair combing and she herself may become increasingly frustrated at his continued dependence upon her for undressing and dressing. In milder cases, there may be difficulty just in tying shoelaces, neckties, sashes and bows, but in more severely afflicted children a true dressing apraxia may make it impossible for the child to put on a coat or dress without some assistance. There may be increasing reliance upon the position of the clothing label in vests, shirts and dresses. The accepted prototype of the young boy returning from school shoeless, bedraggled and unkempt is more acceptable in early than in late primary school. The older child spilling his glass at the meal table or sloshing his food over the tablecloth or his clothing even after it has been cut up for him may present an unacceptable picture to a hungry, irritable father or to self-conscious older siblings inviting a friend to dinner.

By middle childhood, most children are accomplished at a variety of manual activities which may include knitting, sewing, drawing, modelling and general constructional hobbies. A sense of failure and frustration besets the clumsy child who may have to content himself with television despite parental pleas to interest himself more in physical activities. If intellectually inclined he may sublimate these problems by retiring to his bedroom with a book, perhaps to the exclusion of playing ball games with his friends at the park. With the consequent prejudice of his popularity he may be forced to withdraw even further from desirable social contact.

Within the family setting it is usual for the mother first to understand, if not accept, the shortcomings of the child. Often she is placed in the invidious position of having to protect the child from a less tolerant paternal attitude. The father who himself has been a great success in sport is sometimes a lesser hazard than the father who in his youth has failed at sport and embodies his aspirations in an only son. After initial gentle persistence in the attempt to correct the problem, firmer measures tantamount to bullying the child may be employed by the less intelligent parent. The worst reaction the child can evoke from his or her parents is rejection, when extreme compensatory motivation to ingratiate the disinterested parents may be thoroughly thwarted by pure ineptness. Anxiety may well be the healthy reaction of the sensibly involved parent who may devise methods to encourage the child by subterfuge towards improved performance. On the other hand the clumsy child may have to contend with a well-meaning parent who unwittingly pressures the child into swimming or music lessons or to compete in the gymnasium with children of usually average or above average skills.

At school in the classroom the child may be reprimanded constantly for untidy handwriting and drawings. Compulsory sporting and gymnasium periods are anticipated with increasing apprehension and a child may repeatedly invent ingenious excuses such as illness and other indispositions to avoid being the butt of ridicule by his peers. When involved especially in team ball games, his sense of self-deprecation may be heightened by the failure of his team caused by his fumbling and inaccurate throwing. Perhaps his only recourse might be to act the fool as a cover in order that others may think he is not really trying his best; consequently as he gets older he may undersell himself in other spheres of endeavour which may not require physical skills. The truancy record of these children tends to be worse on days when sport is played at school.

A child's self-esteem may be greatly lacking especially if there is a younger, more dexterous sibling who acts as a constant reminder of his own physical ineptitude. He begins to believe that he is 'hopeless' when in fact his anxieties might have been allayed if it were explained to him that he had an intrinsic ineptness through no fault of his own.

Incidence

It has been mentioned previously that as there is a continuum of motor ability in the juvenile population, the point which differentiates 'clumsy' from 'non-clumsy' can only be arbitrary and dependent upon environmental standards. From observations contained in Chapter 4, it is reasonable to assume that at least five per cent of children within the normal school population have significant problems that arise as a result of maladroitness. This figure correlates well with observations by Brenner and Gillman (1966) and Brenner et al (1967).

In the broader context of minimal cerebral dysfunction in which excessive clumsiness is noted as a feature, Paine (1968) stated that currently it was widely maintained that this disorder affected five per cent or more of the entire random child population which would make it the commonest neurological diagnosis among children. Others have put the figure as high as 10 per cent and the prevalence naturally would have depended on the diagnostic criteria which were applied. Clements (1966b) estimated that 5 to 20 per cent and Omenn (1973) that 5 to 15 per cent of the general school population suffered from minimal brain dysfunction which therefore was of major importance in the entire health field. A syndrome which shows considerable overlap with developmental clumsiness, developmental hyperactivity, has an estimated incidence of four per cent in school-age children (Werry, 1968). An apparent increase in the number of children compromised by neurological dysfunctions is often the unintentional aftermath of advances in medical knowledge and care (Clements, 1966a) because of the increasing survival rate in congenital and early acquired encephalopathies.

Of patients with learning disabilities, Minskoff (1973) found that reliably counting the number of learning disabled children in the population appears to be an elusive and difficult task. A national survey of the organisation of instruction to handicapped pupils in the public schools gave an estimate of 2.6 per cent of 45 million pupils in the United States with reported specific learning disabilities (Silverman and Metz, 1973).

Bakwin (1968a) and Reuben and Bakwin (1968) recognised a familial incidence as a characteristic of the developmental disorders where one member of the family might exhibit one or more developmental deviations and others the same or different ones. Clements (1966a) and Paine (1968) maintained that the aberrations of minimal cerebral dysfunction might arise from genetic variations amongst other aetiological factors and Illingworth (1968) also appreciated the importance of familial factors. In related problems such as developmental dysarthria (Morley, Court and Miller, 1954) and developmental dyslexia (Critchley, 1970) a familial tendency is common. Although Pratt (1967) has not recorded a tendency to familial occurrence in 'clumsy children', it should be mentioned that three of the clumsy children in the pilot survey described in Chapter 3 were all from the same sibship and were well known to the Deputy Headmaster for their extreme diffidence towards the sports afternoon when they would frequently develop minor ailments in the attempt to justify their exclusion from this activity.

Although Ford (1966), Bakwin (1968a) and Reuben and Bakwin (1968) recognised a greater incidence of developmental clumsiness in boys than in girls, this observation was not confirmed in the objective analysis detailed in Chapter 4. Perhaps parents tend to become more concerned over their sons than their daughters when there are problems with educational implications and seek advice more readily for their male offspring. However, in allied developmental disorders such as developmental hyperactivity (Werry, 1958), the choreiform syndrome (Wolff and Hurwitz, 1966; Rutter, Graham and Birch, 1966) and developmental dyslexia (Critchley, 1970) a male pro- ponderance is clearly evident.

Any discussion on prevalence or incidence in minimal cerebral dysfunction, or its more specific component syndromes such as developmental clumsiness, must take into consideration the specific age groups which are of relevance. The problems in this context are only of arbitrary practical importance in children between the ages of 6 and 12 years. It is during this age range that manual and other skills should have reached a critical stage of development. In younger age groups, the environment tends to be less reactive and generally kinder because of the wider range of normal variation. Intellectually the older child usually has matured sufficiently to compensate for these problems either by avoidance or concealment.

Aetiology

Aetiological considerations contribute to the understanding of the nature of developmental cerebral dysfunctions, but also have very practical clinical application. Parents are usually motivated by guilt feelings, eugenic planning or simple curiosity to enquire into the cause. Some writers stress an organic basis to the development of the manifestations of 'minimal cerebral dysfunction' in an anatomical sense including perinatal influences which may be responsible for congenital encephalopathy. Others stress the importance of environmental influences, and there are some who favour a disturbance of cerebral integration resulting from a pure defect of neurophysiological development including factors resulting in delayed maturation of the brain. Probably most paediatric neurologists would prefer to think in terms of a multifactorial aetiology.

A basis for anatomical considerations in the causation of developmental apraxia could be interpreted from reports by various authors. McFie, Piercy and Zangwill (1950) suggested that the right occipito-parietal region of the cortex was predominantly involved. It was also thought that apraxia for dressing and the greater part of the constructional disability could be explained in terms of neglect of the left side of visual space. A study by McFie and Zangwill (1960) provided clear documentation that visual-constructive disabilities and right–left disorientation were associated with lesions of the left cerebral hemisphere. "An acquired complex motor ability may be affected by a unilateral lesion without necessarily any disturbance of ideation or any kinetic apraxia" (Langworthy, 1970). Geschwind (1965, 1967) discussed the anatomical disconnection of primary receptive motor areas from one another, in the context of apraxia. Other more general considerations of anatomical disturbance have been given by Knobloch and Pasamanick (1959), Hagberg (1962, 1963), Walshe (1965) and Pincus and Glaser (1966).

Dennis (1941), Pond (1960) and Ellis (1967) have considered particularly the influence of environment in neuropsychiatric disorders. Although deprivation might delay development, it is encouraging that subsequent practice or alteration of environment might rapidly raise the level of achievement up to the level of the child's potential, be it in the motor field or otherwise.

Perinatal pathological influences on development of children have been discussed by Balf (1952), Anderson (1956), Stott (1957), Fraser and Wilks (1959), Prechtl (1960), Steckler (1964) and Collins and Turner (1971). A scientific approach to the evaluation of abnormal perinatal factors has been evolved by Apgar (1953) and Apgar et al (1955), where a newborn infant's status was scored on the basis of performance with respect to five factors including heart rate, respiratory effort, reflex irritability, muscle tone and colour. Kalverboer, Touwen and Prechtl (1973) observed some correlation between minor neurological dysfunctions in the neonatal period and at pre-school-age in children, especially boys. A study by Chase (1973) has shown definite alterations in human brain biochemistry following intra-uterine deprivation, but suggested that these alterations could be recovered with good post-natal care. Sechzer, Faro and Windle (1973) have provided experimental evidence for asphyxia neonatorum as being an important factor in aetiology.

Lilienfeld and Pasamanick (1954) constructed the widely quoted and attractive hypothesis of the 'continuum of reproductive casualty'. According to this theory there is a lethal component of cerebral damage which results in fetal and neonatal deaths and a sub-lethal component which gives rise to a series of clinical and neuropsychiatric syndromes, depending on the degree and location of the damage. They have found that the abnormalities range from the more obvious disabilities of cerebral palsy, epilepsy and mental deficiency through the learning and behavioural difficulties such as reading disability, tics and behaviour disorders of childhood probably as a result of cerebral dis-organisation following minimal brain damage (see also Lilienfeld and Pasamanick, 1955; Pasamanick and Lilienfeld, 1955; Rogers, Lilienfeld and Pasamanick, 1955; Pasamanick and Kawi, 1956; Kawi and Pasamanick, 1958; Knobloch and Pasamanick, 1959). Further parallel contributions have been made by Lord (1937), Luria (1966), Hécaen (1967) and Crichton et al (1971). From personal observations there is strong support to suggest that the clumsiest children are those most likely to have traceable abnormal perinatal influences.

More specifically in relation to perinatal aetiological considerations of developmental clumsiness, Brenner et al (1967), Brenner, Gillman and Farrell (1968) and Edwards (1968) have alluded to the relationship between the physical condition after birth and subsequent performance including motor function. Gesell and Amatruda (1947) described a combination of motor defects including exaggerated extension of the fingers on grasping, peculiar postures of the hands and legs, minor speech defects, mild unsteadiness and generalised clumsiness in young children with histories suggesting birth injury.

Bakwin (1968a) simply stated that the developmental disorders of motility and language were manifestations of inborn alterations in cerebral organisation. No anatomic lesions are demonstrable, nor are there electroencephalographic changes, and it is assumed that the basis is a delay or alteration in the maturation of those areas of the brain that govern motor coordination and language. There have been very strong arguments favouring a confusion in cerebral dominance as the neurophysiological basis of clumsiness or other defects within the spectrum of minimal cerebral palsy. Benson and Geschwind (1968) contended that there appeared to be a rather direct relationship between the maturation of motor skills and the development of cerebral dominance. The child with early strong hand preferences is likely to develop motor activities and fine dexterity earlier than the child with late hand preference; and possibly retarded dominance and clumsiness are related to the same underlying factor. These authors advocated the testing of cerebral dominance acquisition as part of the evaluation of every clumsy child.

Reuben and Bakwin (1968) have considered that failure to establish clearcut lateral dominance or superimposed alterations in lateral dominance may be associated with severe clumsiness. A distinction has been made between the terms ambidextrous, which implies the capability of using both hands with equal dexterity, and ambilevous, where both hands are equally awkward. This concept of the importance of indeterminate cerebral dominance in the production of impaired motor proficiency and other varieties of neurological disability has been supported in discussions by Doll (1951), McFie (1952), Goodglass and Quadfasel (1954), Zangwill (1960b) and Francis-Williams (1963), and is sustained by observations discussed in Chapter 4.

Kinsbourne and Warrington (1962) have favoured the neurophysiological explanation of the basis of developmental disorders. They have propounded that the development of finger sense together with right–left orientation might be regarded as fragments which help to comprise appreciation of the body image. Chalfant and Scheffelin (1969) refer to the integration of cutaneous and kinaesthetic information as 'haptic' processing. It would seem obvious that a child's physical performance would be clumsy if there were a central processing dysfunction of the haptic mechanism of integration. Just as clumsiness can arise from defects of perceptual development, so can perceptual development be hindered in the child who cannot physically manipulate objects or in whom the peripheral sensory system is not intact (Isom, 1966).

The term 'minimal cerebral damage' (Paine, 1968) implies that organic problems underlie the manifestations of the encephalopathy. These aberrations may arise from genetic variation, biochemical irregularities, perinatal brain insults, illnesses or injuries sustained during the years critical for the development and maturation of the central nervous system, or from unknown causes. Amongst those who have discussed a biochemical aetiology, Wender (1971, 1973) has suggested a defect of monoamine metabolism in minimal brain dysfunction. The neurological implications of widespread subclinical lead intoxication have been discussed by Needleman (1973). Most authors, when challenged about the concept of structural versus primary physiological aetiology, would probably yield to the concept of multiple factors, sometimes with varying emphasis on a particular syndrome. Thus, where familial or genetic factors play an important part, it might be assumed that a physiological basis is applicable, but against this one must also appreciate that anatomical variation of the brain (which may not be apparent histologically) could equally have a genetic basis. Authors who have considered a multi-factorial or heterogeneous aetiology are Ingram (1963), Walton (1963), Rodin, Lucas and Simon (1964), Clements (1966a), Critchley (1968a), Illingworth (1968) and Omenn (1973).

Illingworth (1971) has strongly decried the use of the terms 'brain damage' and 'birth injury' because parental distress could be caused through the implication of blame for the obstetrician or the midwife, and the diagnosis was usually wrong in any case. Even if the words 'damage' or 'injury' were applicable, they should be avoided meticulously unless accurate, as in cases of head injury, encephalitis or meningitis occurring in the newborn period.

Cerebral immaturity in aetiology

Werner and Kaplan (1963) have defined maturation as the process of growth from unstable and primitive to stable and highly integrated hierarchic behaviour. In discussing the principles of learning, Harlow and Harlow (1962) have recognised progressive improvement which is independent of special experience because of the effect of maturation and not of learning by practice. Illingworth (1968) has propounded the theory that delayed motor development as a familial feature presumably may be due to a familial pattern of late myelination. Wernicke (1874) gave credence to the importance of progressive connections between different parts of the brain in the emergence of complex activities. He asserted that complex activities were learned by means of connections between a small number of functional regions which dealt with the primary motor and sensory activities.

Maturational lag has been offered as a basic explanation for developmental clumsiness (Annell, 1949; *British Medical Journal,* 1962; Bakwin, 1968a) and a similar view has been expressed for cases of developmental dyslexia (Critchley, 1967, 1968a, 1970; Cohn, 1961b). Klapper (1966) has warned against the emphasis attached to the concept of maturational lag, a term which supposes a permissible wide range of early achievement to be 'normal' for a given child and which requires only the passage of time for correction to a more favourable 'norm'. With respect to reading, for example, whereas significant progress might be expected by the end of the second grade, a marked discrepancy between the developmental progress of the individual child and that of his age-matched group prior to this stage should be sufficient cause for investigation. In discussing neurodevelopmental lag with particular reference to the motor component of the nervous system, Kinsbourne (1973) stated that sometimes it was inconsequential to the child's daily life and social adjustment, such as when it involved some minor reflex abnormality. At other times, it might be of major importance, such as when a motor inadequacy rendered the child clumsy. Associated movements have been regarded as a major index of motor immaturity, contributing to the 'clumsy child' syndrome, but their use in diagnosis is complicated by the difficulty in establishing clear-cut criteria for their occurrence. Ayres (1972a), in discussing developmental apraxia, considers that there must be dysfunction in vestibular and other proprioceptive mechanisms which would contribute to the symptoms of postural and bilateral integration disorders in apraxic children. She has also described praxis as a learned ability to plan and direct a temporal series of co-ordinated movements towards achieving a result—usually a skilled and non-habitual act. It is the end product of a developmental process involving afferent synthesis of the entire post-ontogenetic experience.

Manifestations of Abnormal Behaviour and Emotional Problems

There are two basic reasons why a child with a chronic encephalopathy might exhibit a disorder of behaviour. Firstly, the organic disturbance of cerebral function could directly influence behaviour and emotional responses through a lack of integrity of neural pathways concerned with emotion. Secondly, an emotional disturbance could develop from the child's own frustrations through repeated failure and resentment over rejection by parents and teachers.

It has been stressed repeatedly by virtually all writers on the subject of minimal cerebral dysfunction and developmental clumsiness that one of the first considerations in management should be to ease the emotional burden on the afflicted children. A full but simple explanation to the child and to his parents, and if necessary a modification of his educational programme, may be all that is necessary to dispel undue anxiety. In fact the emotional overlay may dominate the clinical picture to such an extent that the child may be brought to the doctor because of behavioural symptoms rather than the primary difficulty (Bakwin, 1968a). Some children can be so emotionally disturbed that they cannot be adequately taught in an ordinary school (Dare and Gordon, 1970). By the time they reach school they often have already developed disturbed patterns of behaviour at home because of being clumsy, uncontrolled and unco-ordinated and they frequently exhibit restlessness and distractibility (Francis-Williams, 1963). The child's associated overactivity, impulsiveness and defective concentration causes considerable difficulty at school, particularly if a child is thought by the teacher to be just naughty (Illingworth, 1968). The child with disturbances of visual perception may be excluded from games because he is clumsy, derided because he seems ill-mannered at the dinner table, scolded because his writing is a mere scribble, or treated with visible worry or anger by his parents because he cannot read. Such a child soon feels himself excluded and rejected, leading to feelings of inadequacy, depression, aggression and further disruption of his environment (Frostig, 1963; Köng, 1963).

Some of the parental responses to a handicapped child discussed by Michel (1963) include shock with disappointment, denial ('he is not severely or permanently handicapped'), guilt, disturbed marital relationship because of neglect of the father by the mother or neglect of a healthy sibling, and hostility towards the child. Amongst the specific problems that have been described are truancy (Annell, 1949), unpopularity with peers, and rejection by adults (Brenner and Gillman, 1966). Further observations on maladjustment and disturbed emotions are made by Brenner et al (1967), Brenner and Gillman (1968) and Reuben and Bakwin (1968). Headache may develop in response to various stresses at school (Knight et al, 1962; Thetford, Schulman and Farmer, 1967).

Although emotional disturbance is frequently caused by academic failure, it may itself contribute to a child's lack of success at school, because the maladjusted child performs less well as a result of restlessness, distractibility, resistance to discipline, antisocial conduct and negative responses from teachers. Thus the motivation of the child is likely to wane even further and the chances of academic success become even more remote (Wolff, 1969). The psychological aspects of encephalopathy have been discussed fully by Floyer (1955), Bradley (1957), Eisenberg (1957), Taylor (1959), Pond (1960), Teuber and Rudel (1962), Clements (1966a) and Conners (1967).

Delayed Speech and Speech Problems

Mental retardation is the most frequent cause of delayed speech (Bakwin, 1968b). Brain (1961) defined developmental disorders of speech as those conditions in which acquisition of speech was retarded or abnormal as the result of abnormality in the central nervous system at birth, but in practice excluding gross mental defect and embracing only an isolated abnormality of speech which had not been conditioned by psychological causes, hearing loss and disturbed organs of speech. The disorders due to neurological dysfunction include developmental dysarthria and developmental articulatory apraxia (Morley, 1957). The distinction between these two categories is in the disturbance of central nervous system integration, which is higher in the effector pathways in developmental articulatory apraxia, and unlike developmental dysarthria is not associated with apraxia of the tongue and palate. Thus it is misleading to assume that speech disorders are similar in the different types of cerebral palsy (Morley, Court and Miller, 1954; Morely et al, 1955; Ingram, 1964). Varying types of speech defect seem to occur with greater frequency in clumsy children (Walton, Ellis and Court, 1962; Brenner et al, 1967; Reuben and Bakwin, 1968).

School and Educational Problems

With the children described here, many aspects of formal school education can be disturbed both in the classroom and on the sports field. The educational problems are usually due to the combined effect of the basic cerebral dysfunction and emotional overlay. Children with learning disabilities of varying types have been classified within the ambit of minimal cerebral dysfunction or developmental cerebral dysfunction. The National Advisory Committee on Handicapped Children (1967) developed the following definition as a clarification of the identity of children with learning disabilities:

"Children with special learning disabilities exhibit a disorder in one or more of the basic psychological processes involved in understanding or using spoken or written language. These may be manifested in disorders of listening, thinking, talking, reading, writing, spelling or arithmetic. They include conditions which have been referred to as perceptual handicaps, brain injury, minimal brain dysfunction, dyslexia, developmental aphasia, etc. They do not include learning problems which are due primarily to visual, hearing or motor handicaps, to mental retardation, emotional disturbance or environmental disadvantage."

Certain arbitrary standards of achievement are most rigidly applied during school years where there is intensive comparative evaluation. Within this system, children frequently do not measure up to expectations, but there is now an increasing awareness that many children with normal intelligence still exhibit peculiarities of their mental processes which interfere with their ability to attain certain standard educational requirements (Masland, 1969a). The very comprehensive report on central processing dysfunctions in children under the auspices of the National Institute of Neurological Diseases and Stroke embodied a review of scientific knowledge regarding the learning disabilities of children with minimal cerebral dysfunction.

Organic brain syndromes with evidence of overt motor defect (cerebral palsy) are extremely common and are one of the major considerations in the educational management of children attending cerebral palsy centres. Apraxia can be disruptive to both central organisation and discriminative learning (Woods, 1957; Berko, 1966). Learning disabilities in less severe chronic organic brain syndromes are of similar nature and are generally milder, although a major isolated learning defect may occur in the presence of congenital encephalopathy which might be identifiable only collaterally by 'soft neurological signs' or electroencephalographic changes. Poor educational performance in this context is discussed by Thelander, Phelps and Kirk (1958), Prechtl and Stemmer (1962) and Boshes and Myklebust (1964). Brenner and her associates (Brenner and Gillman, 1966; Brenner et al, 1967; Brenner, Gillman and Farrell, 1968), Bakwin (1968a) and Frostig (1971) make special reference to the learning difficulties in clumsy children. Emphasis on the aspect of learning disability in children with minimal cerebral dysfunction is made by Clements (1966a), Kirk (1968), Gallagher et al (1969) and Bateman and Schiefelbusch (1969).

Electroencephalography

In the author's view, electroencephalography can make only a minor diagnostic contribution because of its apparent lack of specificity relating to abnormalities observed within the context of minimal cerebral dysfunction. It has served mainly in the statistical sphere where correlations may be found between increased (and usually non-specific) EEG abnormality and these minor neurological defects. The increased frequency of abnormality observed in clumsy children, especially in children with minimal cerebral dysfunction, must support the aetiological contention of a basic underlying encephalopathy; and a clear-cut, focal EEG abnormality would probably carry as much weight in organic implication as a focal neurological sign.

The EEG has also been described as an important but frequently misused supplement to the neurological examination (Miller, 1969). But a fraction of the brain's total activity is reflected through the electrodes which commonly cover only about one-third of the brain, and paroxysmal disturbances may not be manifest during the 20 minutes or so of routine recording time in any one patient. There are many variables which make EEG interpretation difficult; these include the patient's age and state of consciousness and the recording technique. The very large number of variables and the gross fundamental complexity of electroencephalography necessitate an undue subjective element in EEG interpretation which is likely to lead to bias.

In defining developmental disorders of motility and language as manifestations of inborn alterations of cerebral organisation, Bakwin (1968a) has included as a sine qua non that there are no demonstrable anatomical lesions, nor are there EEG changes. However, in the usually accepted sense of developmental cerebral dysfunction, whether or not 'damage' is implied or unlikely, most surveys have revealed that a higher proportion of EEG abnormalities are recorded from these children than in the general juvenile population. The abnormalities that may be present in 50 per cent or more of cases are less often spike-wave complexes or seizure discharges than merely lesser disorders of rate, amplitude and rhythm (Paine, 1968). The EEG abnormalities are usually minor and do not normally contribute to the practical management of the child in any way. Although there may be a significant degree of interrelationship between neurological and EEG abnormalities in children more severely affected (Annett, Lee and Ounsted, 1961), Paine, Werry and Quay (1968) in a study of 83 children felt that this observation could not be extrapolated to cases of minimal cerebral dysfunction. Further shortcomings of EEG appraisal are discussed by Glaser (1963) and Kiloh and Osselton (1961). Critchley (1970) has not been impressed with EEG changes in this disorder and allied problems. Observations by Hanvick (1953), Chorost, Spivack and Levine (1959), Benton and Bird (1963) and Davidoff and Johnson (1964) should probably be interpreted with caution.

Satterfield (1973) and Satterfield et al (1973) reported a study of auditory evoked cortical responses in 31 children with minimal brain dysfunction and 21 control subjects. Evoked cortical potentials in the experimental group had significantly lower amplitudes and longer latencies that those in the control group. These findings suggested a neurophysiological basis for minimal brain dysfunction consistent with a theory of delayed maturation of the central nervous system.

Despite its limitations, the role of electroencephalography in the management of clumsy children or others with minimal cerebral dysfunction should not be neglected and should probably be reserved for the following indications:

1. Suspicion of epilepsy, such as brief episodes of apparent day-dreaming or loss of awareness of surroundings, impulsive behaviour, or paroxysmal stereotyped episodes of abnormal behaviour. It is obviously an attractive hypothesis that paroxysmal discharges in the EEG, even if not associated

with any visible abnormal movement, might reflect breaks in the train of thought or lapses of attention and thus interfere with learning (Paine, 1965).
2. Suspicion of a progressive neurological condition.
3. Confirmation of a focal abnormality as suggested by neurological observation.
4. Reassurance.

Management and Prognosis

The assessment and the overall management of the clumsy child are discussed in Chapters 5 and 6. Factors relating to history, examination and special testing are treated in full and the diagnosis and differential diagnosis are considered. Particular attention is paid to educational aspects both in the classroom and on the sporting field, and to the role of remediation. It is encouraging that longitudinal studies in this disorder tend to show a favourable outcome for the child. Full documentation of the factors of prognosis are discussed in the conclusion of the final chapter.

CHAPTER THREE

An Investigation of 21 Children with Developmental Clumsiness

This aspect of the investigation was carried out at the Regional Neurological Centre and Royal Victoria Infirmary in Newcastle upon Tyne, England. The children in the study had all been referred for assessment at the Percy Hedley Centre which functions as a school, clinic and workshop for handicapped children with cerebral palsy. The findings in these children have been presented and discussed previously by Gubbay et al (1965). The children had presented over a period of some years from various random sources of referral in the North of England and in Scotland. The basic abnormality which required further consideration in all the subjects was severe clumsiness which was sufficient to interfere significantly with their ordinary daily motor activity. It was recognised at the outset that these children did not have cerebral palsy in the usual sense, but in general their lack of motor facility was as incapacitating to them as in cases of cerebral palsy. The main point of differentiation from other children referred to the Centre was the absence or paucity of physical signs, especially those usually associated with defects within the pyramidal or extrapyramidal systems. It was this study which prompted the idea to develop standardised tests which would help to recognise clumsy children more rapidly and with greater precision. It also stimulated the need for further detailed delineation of the clinical characteristics of the clumsier child in the community, when correlations with other developmental factors, family history, and broad environmental influences could be forthcoming.

At the time of the study, it was appreciated that various types of apraxia and agnosia of congenital origin or arising in infancy might occur in isolation and might be quite dissociated from any other collateral clinical evidence of brain dysfunction such as amentia, spastic weakness or involuntary movements. The lack of dexterity in children with overt 'cerebral palsy' was known to receive abundant sympathetic understanding and practical attention from parents, teachers and educational authorities. Special provision often was made automatically for their education and management which admittedly demanded greater skill and patience than was the case in normal children. By contrast, the clumsy child with no overt neurological signs was less easily recognised and usually received less sympathy and understanding; hence he became more diffident in attempting manual skills and was often accused in turn of laziness or misbehaviour or suspected of being mentally dull. The natural outcome was a feeling of frustration, often leading to a behaviour disorder which aggravated the child's problems of learning and performance (De la Cruz and LaVeck, 1965). Thus, Wolff (1969) had found diminishing motivation of maladjusted children which made the chances of academic success even more remote.

MATERIALS AND METHODS

This chapter deals with the study of 21 children who presented with an intrinsic clumsiness resulting in defective performance of skills which depend upon manual dexterity and bodily agility. They all had normal intelligence as defined by a Verbal IQ exceeding 80 in the Wechsler Intelligence Scale for Children (WISC). Four of these children were reported previously (Walton, 1961; Walton, Ellis and Court, 1962) and some follow-up information concerning these cases is provided. A detailed inquiry was made into the antenatal, perinatal and developmental history of all cases as well as into associated and past illnesses. Hand, foot and eye dominance were determined and assessments were made of language function including speech, reading and writing. The Reading Quotient

$$\frac{\text{Reading Age}}{\text{Chronological Age}} \times 100$$

was estimated from Reading Attainment Test RI (Schonell and Schonell, 1950), and the ability to calculate was checked against the Arithmetic Subscore obtained from the WISC. Appreciation of body image and ex-trapersonal space was assessed by testing right—left orientation, finger sense (including the 'In-Between' test of Kinsbourne and Warrington, 1962), simultaneous bilateral cutaneous and visual stimuli, tactile localisation and the drawing of a clock-face and maps where applicable. Tests were carried out for visual object agnosia, simultagnosia (failure to recognise the meaning of a picture as a whole although the details are correctly appreciated) and colour agnosia. The presence or absence of tactile agnosia or astereognosis and graphaesthesia was determined.

Apraxias of ideational, ideomotor and motor (limb-kinetic) type were tested by asking the child to perform complicated tasks (e.g. folding a sheet of newspaper and placing it in an envelope), a series of organised movements such as waving goodbye, making a fist, etc. and to demonstrate the use of objects such as a comb, toothbrush and spoon. The child was also asked to copy from the examiner random positions of the fingers and hands in space on his left and right sides independently. Facial and lingual apraxia were recognised by the inability to move the face and tongue according to command. Constructional apraxia was demonstrated by the inability to copy simple geometric designs with matchsticks, or by drawing, and the inability to fit a series of objects of various shapes into appropriate slots. Dressing apraxia was recognised by observing the child while he was undressing and dressing before and after the complete neurological and general examination which was carried out in every case. Electroencephalographic (EEG) recordings were taken in each case.

In all, 24 selected children whose presenting symptom was severe clumsiness were reviewed (Table 3.1). Three children were excluded from further consideration when their clumsiness was found to be due solely to pyramidal or extrapyramidal disease. The remaining 21 children who exhibited varying degrees and types of apraxia and agnosia (Cases 1 to 21 inclusive) were further subdivided into two groups. Group I (cases 1 to 14) comprised 14 children with apraxia and/or agnosia in isolation, while Group II (cases 15 to 21) contained children whose difficulties were primarily due to similar executive or cognitive defects, but in whom were found minimal evidence of dysfunction in pyramidal or cerebellar pathways, insufficient to contribute significantly to their fundamental clumsiness. Three cases were included in Group II because the children in question had suffered major cerebral illnesses in the past.

Table 3.1. Clinical subdivision of all cases examined

Group		No. of cases
Group I[a] :	Apraxia and agnosia only	14 (Case Nos. 1–14)
Group II[a] :	Apraxia and agnosia with pyramidal signs, cerebellar signs or past cerebral illness	7 (Case Nos. 15–21)
	Pyramidal or extrapyramidal signs only	3
	Total	24

[a] See Table 3.3 for further analysis of Groups I and II.
Reproduced with the kind permission of the editor of *Brain*.

The Examination Proforma

All the children referred for the study were subjected to a standardised individual assessment proforma. The children were all accompanied by at least one parent and were each examined personally. After several children had been examined it became obvious that a number of items in the proforma were unsatisfactory and these are not detailed here. Wherever possible the electroencephalograms were performed on the same day as the clinical assessment. All of the children had been assessed previously at the Percy Hedley Centre, Newcastle upon Tyne. They were now referred for detailed comprehensive examination including all parameters related to developmental clumsiness. The proforma (with commentary) is shown below.

DEVELOPMENTAL APRAXIA AND AGNOSIA—PROFORMA

Reference:

Name
Date of Birth
Sex
Home Address

Consultant
General Practitioner
Hospital Number
Present History Relating to Clumsiness:

Special Physical Ineptitudes:

Obstetric History and Neonatal Period:

Mother's health in pregnancy
Period of gestation
Duration of labour
Complications of labour (including APH and injury)
Type of delivery
Place of delivery
Birth weight
Onset of respirations
Jaundice or cyanosis
Neonatal condition and treatment

Previous Obstetric History and Family History:

No. of abortions—dates and causes
No. of stillbirths—dates and causes
Neonatal deaths—dates and causes
Maternal present age and health
Paternal present age and health
Siblings (in order)—name, age and health
1.
2.
3.
4.
5.
6.
7.
8.
Other relevant family history

Developmental Milestones

Sat unaided
Crawled
Walked unaided
Words
Sentences
Diurnal and nocturnal continence

Began to read
Began to write
Drank unaided from cup
Fed unaided with knife, fork and spoon
Began using doorknobs and doorhandles
Able to completely dress and undress
(a) buttons (b) bows (c) ties
Brushed hair
Cleaned teeth
Rode tricycle
Rode bicycle
Cricket
Football

Associated Diseases and Past History:

PRESENT EXAMINATION

Date of examination
Age
General inspection
Co-operation
Mood
General activity
Skull contour
Skull circumference
Gait
Running
Jumping
Hopping, left and right foot

Hemisphere dominance:

Manual dominance
Ocular dominance
Pedal dominance
Interpretation of ambiguous figures

(Manual dominance was assessed by determining which hand was used for writing, combing the hair, brushing the teeth and catching and throwing a ball. Eye dominance was tested by determining the fixing eye used by the subject looking at a distant object through a hole in a card about 30 cm away from the open eyes. Visual hemisphere dominance was estimated by the use of the ambiguous figure by McFie (1952). Footedness was assessed by determining which leg was most consistently used to kick a ball.)

Speech:

Description of speech and formulation
Description of articulation

Naming of common objects

(The subject was presented with 10 common objects for visual identification.)

Understanding of commands:

'Walk over to the couch and touch the pillow!'
'Walk backwards to the washbasin and touch the soap!'
'Hop to the door and touch the doorhandle!'
'When I put my hand in my pocket, but not before, close your eyes and poke out your tongue!'

Reading aloud:

Schonell's Reading Test RI (Schonell and Schonell, 1950).

Writing to dictation:

(The patients were asked to write their names and addresses and the following dictation: 'my cat likes to play all day', and 'the quick brown fox jumps over the lazy dog'. The subject also had to write all digits from 1 to 10.)

Calculation:

Addition
Subtraction
Multiplication
Division

(Each child was subjected to the same mental arithmetic proforma, which is not reproduced here because it was self-styled and only used as an approximate assessment. A more accurate standardised assessment was forthcoming from the arithmetic subscore of the Verbal WISC Test.)

Body Image and Extrapersonal Space:

Right–left orientation:

'which is your right hand?'
'which is your left hand?'
'which is my right hand?'
'which is my left hand?'
The examiner then turned around, crossed the hands and said:
'which is my right hand?'
'which is my left hand?'

Simultaneous bilateral visual stimuli
Simultaneous bilateral cutaneous stimuli

Drawing of clock-face and numbers
Drawing of map of England inserting London and Newcastle

Gnosis:

Interpretation of simple pictures

(The subject was presented with three line drawings from Binet Test Cards A, B and C and asked to describe the picture and what it was meant to convey. This was used as a test of visual agnosia and also of simultagnosia, i.e. the ability to understand the picture as a whole although unable to appreciate details.)

Recognition of individual fingers on self and examiner

(The examiner named each finger on his own hand and then asked the subject to name his or her own fingers in turn. The 'in-between' test was explained to the patient in detail (Kinsbourne and Warrington, 1962) and a few trials were done with the patient's eyes open. The subject then closed the eyes and the test was performed on each hand separately. If the patient made more than two errors he was designated as having finger agnosia.)

Stereognosis

(Using same test objects as for nominal aphasia.)

Graphaesthesia

(Figures were drawn on the patient's right and left forefingers respectively in the correct position for the subject. To do this one had to stand beside the patient and face in the same direction. An occasional error or mild misinterpretation such as six for zero was passed.)

Praxis:

Use of (a) comb
     (b) scissors
     (c) toothbrush
     (d) knife and fork

(These four test objects were handed to the patient in turn and the performance was noted—for ideomotor apraxia.)

'Fold sheet of notepaper and place in envelope!'

(Ideational apraxia)

'Make a fist!'
'Clap your hands!'
'Snap your fingers!'
'Scratch your head!'
'Put out your tongue!'
'Close your eyes!'
'Wink!'
'Blow a kiss!'

'Salute!'   (Ideomotor apraxia)
'Wave goodbye!'
'Pretend to knock at a door!'
'Pretend to count out money!'
'Pretend to play a piano!'
'Construction of match model'   (The subject was asked to copy con-
                                             structions of a triangle, square and cube.)

Posting box   (The subject was asked to place various
                                             objects of differing size and shape into
                                             appropriate slots.)

Draw a house
Draw a daisy
Dressing and undressing
Fastening buttons
Tying shoelaces

ROUTINE PHYSICAL EXAMINATION

Cranial Nerves:

Motor System:
Development
Wasting
Abnormal movements
Posture
Tone
Power
Co-ordination:
   Finger-nose test
   Fine finger movement
   Rapid alternating movement
   Heel, knee, shin test
   Rapid foot movement

Reflexes:

            R   L
JJ
BJ
SJ
TJ
Abdo U
Abdo L
KJ
AJ
Plantars
Sensation:
Cottonwool

Pinprick
Vibration
Joint position sense
Two-point discrimination

General Examination

Congenital Abnormalities:
Height
Weight
EEG   (All the EEGs were interpreted by one observer, Dr. D. D. Barwick. No control EEGs were carried out and there were no sleep recordings.)

THE CONTROLS

Of the 21 subjects who were fully investigated, 13 were male and 8 female. The age range at the time of assessment was between 9 years 5 months and 17 years 4 months (mean 12 years 6 months). Although most of the abnormal findings in these cases were gross and obvious, it was considered wise to submit a control group of children to a limited battery of tests. The controls (see Table 3.2) comprised 10 normal schoolchildren of average capabilities as judged by a headmistress who selected them at random from an average class. The age range in this group was 9 years 10 months to 10 years 2 months (mean 10 years) with WISC full scale scores varying from 94 to 128 (mean 113). None of these control patients showed any evidence of ideational,

Table 3.2. Observations made on 10 school children (controls)

Control No.	1	2	3	4	5	6	7	8	9	10
Age (years)	$10\frac{1}{12}$	10	10	10	$10\frac{1}{12}$	$9\frac{10}{12}$	$10\frac{2}{12}$	$9\frac{11}{12}$	$10\frac{2}{12}$	10
Sex	F	F	F	M	F	F	F	F	F	M
Manual dominance	R	R	R	R	R	R	R	R	R	R
Crossed laterality	−	−	−	+	−	+	−	−	−	−
R−L disorientation	−	±	−	−	−	−	±	−	−	−
Finger agnosia	−	−	−	±	−	−	+	−	−	−
Astereognosis	−	−	−	−	−	−	−	−	−	−
Ideational apraxia	−	−	−	−	−	−	−	−	−	−
Ideomotor apraxia	−	−	−	−	−	−	−	−	−	−
Constructional apraxia	±	−	−	−	−	−	+	−	−	−
Writing abnormality	−	−	−	−	−	−	±	−	−	−
Topographical agnosia	−	−	−	−	−	−	−	−	−	−
Abnormal movements	−	−	−	−	−	−	−	−	−	−
WISC Performance IQ	99	99	122	103	135	114	89	117	103	118
WISC Verbal IQ	103	119	118	114	116	111	100	111	125	118
WISC Full Scale IQ	101	110	122	109	128	114	94	115	116	120

The overall differences between Verbal and Performance IQ are not significant.
Reproduced with the kind permission of the editor of *Brain*.

ideomotor or motor apraxia or of topographical agnosia or abnormal movements. One of them was found to have a combination of mild right—left confusion and moderate finger agnosia and constructional apraxia. One child had a mild right—left confusion, one a mild finger agnosia and another a mild constructional apraxia. All the other children showed no abnormality. As the control group fell in the lower range of the mental age of the clumsy children, it may be safely assumed that most of the anomalies of recognition and performance observed in the clumsy children were in fact valid abnormalities and could not have been construed as being within the range of normal reactions in children of comparable or even lower mental age.

It should be noted from Table 3.2 that all of the four control children with abnormalities had higher Verbal scores than Performance scores and that there was only one other control child with such a disparity between Verbal and Performance scores. All the children with equal or higher Performance scores than Verbal scores showed no abnormalities on these tests. The results of the tests were fully tabulated before the IQ figures were available from the psychologist in order to reduce observer bias.

CASE REPORTS

Group I

Case 1

Summary. Male aged 12 years. Thought to be mentally retarded when first starting school. He had untidy writing, constructional apraxia and was slow in learning to dress and undress, comb hair and brush teeth. WISC Verbal IQ 116, Performance IQ 93, Reading Quotient 98. EEG immature with mild focal abnormality.

Report. C.H., the elder of two children, was originally thought at the age of 4 years to be less agile than most children of his age. After starting school at the age of 5 years he was suspected of being mentally retarded and the only abnormality on neurological examination was a disorder of movement suggesting chorea. Intelligence testing at the age of 6 years 3 months using the WISC gave a Verbal score of 137 and Performance score of 97. He was unable to construct models with blocks, sticks or matches or to fit objects of variable shape into appropriate holes. His writing was slow and clumsy with frequent reversals.

It was only by the age of 9 years that he was capable of dressing and undressing himself, brushing his hair and cleaning his teeth unassisted, and had begun to lose the tendency to difficult and aggressive behaviour. His intelligence test (WISC) was repeated at 11 years and on this occasion the Verbal score was 116 and Performance score 93.

Detailed assessment at 12 years 2 months revealed that he was clumsy in hopping on either foot. He was right-handed but left-footed. The Reading Quotient was 98 and when writing to dictation he moved his pencil clumsily and slowly to produce untidy but legible writing with no spelling errors or reversals. There was a moderate degree of right—left confusion and he was unable to construct a match design of a cube or to draw one adequately. He now had difficulty in dressing and undressing. No abnormal movements were evident at this examination and the rest of the physical examination was negative.

The EEG showed a slight excess of right-sided posterior slow activity with greater asymmetry during hyperventilation and one paroxysmal burst of delta over the whole left hemisphere suggesting a slight suspicion of left-sided pathology.

Case 2

Summary. Male aged 16 years. Four weeks premature after surgical induction for eclampsia and birth weight 2.0 kg. Speech disturbed after tonsillitis aged 18 months. Clumsy since early childhood. Difficulty in imitating movements of lips and tongue with developmental dysarthria. Poor handwriting and constructional apraxia with gradual improvement. WISC Verbal IQ 120, Performance IQ 106, Reading age 14 years 5 months. EEG immature with left temporal abnormality.

Report. D.L., the elder of two children, was born 1 month prematurely following surgical induction for eclampsia and in spite of a birth weight of 2.0 kg he made good progress, sitting at 7 months and walking at 1 year. By 15 months he was using words and phrases, but at 18 months he had a severe attack of tonsillitis without apparent neurological complications and did not begin to speak easily again until his fourth year.

From early childhood he had been regarded as clumsy; he seemed to know what he wanted to do, but was unable to make his hands perform the necessary action. When examined at the age of 12 years, his gait and all the movements of his limbs were excessively clumsy. When he was tested on the WISC his Verbal score was 99 and his Performance score was 86. He had considerable difficulty in imitating movements as in pursing his lips and putting out his tongue. His speech was still slow, slurred and indistinct, many words were incorrectly pronounced, but there was no lack of language. Repetitive opposition of the thumb and of individual fingers in turn was very poorly performed; his handwriting was crude and the letters ill-formed. He was unable to construct models or to place shaped objects in the appropriate holes.

On assessment at the age of 16 years and 11 months he was right-handed, right-eyed and right-footed. His speech was now greatly improved although he often mispronounced the letters 's' and 'v'. His Reading Age* was estimated to be 14 years 5 months. Handwriting was untidy, but otherwise unremarkable. He now showed no constructional or dressing difficulty and his drawings seemed quite adequate. There was some difficulty in copying finger postures with his hands, particularly on the left side, and he had similar trouble with

---

* Reading Quotients were not estimated when the chronological age exceeded 15 years.

complex tongue movements. Tone was diminished in the upper and lower limbs. The deep tendon reflexes were brisk, abdominal reflexes were present and the plantar responses were flexor. Fine finger movements were well executed on this occasion. A recent reassessment of his WISC gave a Verbal score of 120 and a Performance score of 106.

The EEG showed a marked degree of immaturity with right posterior temporal delta activity and some left posterior temporal sharp waves accentuated after hyperventilation. The appearances were suggestive of a left temporal structural abnormality.

Case 3

Summary. Male aged 13 years. Eight weeks premature, birth weight 1.6 kg, neonatal difficulty, slow motor milestones and speech development. Often thought to be mentally defective. Nystagmoid eye movements. Late with manual development, ungainly gait, dysarthric speech, impaired finger sense, graphaesthesia and stereoanaesthesia. Apraxia of limbs, impaired two-point discrimination. Verbal IQ 95, Performance IQ 78, Reading Quotient 100. EEG suggested right posterior focal epileptogenic lesion.

Report. D.N., the oldest child in a family of three, was born 8 weeks prematurely and his birth weight was 1.6 kg. He was cyanosed after birth and sucked poorly for the first 2 weeks of life. He sat up at 1 year and walked at the age of $2\frac{1}{4}$ years. Although he used sentences at $2\frac{1}{2}$ years, speech was indistinct and almost unintelligible. From an early age it had been noted that movements of his limbs, and particularly of his hands, were extremely clumsy. With speech therapy from the age of 6 years his speech improved and at that age he was able to read, but writing and drawing remained extremely poor. Although he had often been judged to be mentally defective, his WISC scores at the age of 8 years were 105 Verbal and 82 Performance, and when later estimated they were 95 Verbal and 78 Performance respectively. It was noted that his parents had always observed persistent nystagmoid eye movements and he always seemed to have difficulty in judging heights and distances or in seeing anything that was not immediately ahead so that he tended to stumble frequently in unfamiliar surroundings. Between the ages of 2 and 10 years he had four generalised seizures but none had occurred following the introduction of 30 mg of phenobarbitone twice daily.

At the age of 13 years 5 months he still was clumsy in the manipulation of such objects as knife and fork and doorhandles and it was only in the previous year or so that he had learned to dress and undress himself and brush his hair. His gait was stooped and gangling and he was unsteady when trying to hop on either foot. He was right-handed and right-footed for most activities but was left-eyed. Articulation was marred by defective pronunciation of several consonants and was associated with a facial and lingual apraxia. His Reading Quotient was 100, but reading was slow because of impaired visual acuity associated with a coarse nystagmus which was present in all directions. Similarly visual identification of objects and picture symbols was tardy although eventually accurate. Despite full orientation for right and left he sometimes perceived that the examiner was touching both hands when his eyes were closed although only the right side was being touched. He exhibited very poor finger sense which was much worse on the left side of his body and also had a predominantly left-sided graphaesthesia with profound bilateral stereo-anaesthesia. Ideational and ideomotor apraxia were demonstrable and he was unable to imitate certain simple postures of the examiner's fingers and arms. Although slow in the execution of tests to demonstrate constructional apraxia, he was eventually quite accurate. Examination of the motor system was negative but the threshold of two-point discrimination was increased to 3 cm in both forefingers and joint position sense was moderately impaired in the toes and fingers bilaterally.

High-voltage spike discharges were noted in the right posterior parietal region of the EEG and these were rhythmical outbursts associated with slow activity. Hyperventilation and photic stimulation increased the prominence of the spike discharges. The appearances suggested the presence of a right posterior focal epileptogenic lesion.

Case 4

Summary. Female aged 11 years. Congenital pulmonary stenosis and slow speech development. Great difficulty in learning to read and write and slow with motor skills. Sinistral with right–left confusion, finger agnosia, graphaesthesia, apraxia, constructional apraxia. WISC Verbal IQ 104, Performance IQ 71, Reading Quotient 80. EEG suggested diencephalic disturbance of epileptic type.

Report. J.M., a girl with congenital pulmonary stenosis, was the second of five children. She was born, after a gestational period of 38 weeks, by normal delivery and her birth weight was 2.5 kg. Although she did not speak until the age of $2\frac{1}{2}$ years, her motor development was not retarded. When she first attended school her parents were aware of her lack of physical and manual skills and in particular she had great difficulty in learning to write. She was unable to ride a tricycle until the age of 6 years or to dress and undress until she was 8 years old.

When examined at the age of 11 years 9 months, she was still unable to tie her shoelaces or necktie or to insert a slide into her hair. She was left-handed, left-footed and right-eyed and her Reading Quotient was 80. There was a mild right–left confusion with severe bilateral finger agnosia and some graphaesthesia of the right hand. She could not demonstrate how she would use an imaginary pair of scissors and had difficulty in copying simple postures of the examiner's limbs with her own limbs. The presence of a constructional apraxia was demonstrated and on completion of the neurological examination no further abnormality could be found. The WISC gave a Verbal score of 104 and Performance score of 71.

The EEG was basically a grossly unstable, polyrhythmic record with a great deal of posteriorly disposed delta activity and occasionally increased slow activity over the right hemisphere. Photic stimulation induced a generalised outburst of slow waves and spike discharges. The appearances were those of a fairly gross instability together with evidence of a diencephalic disturbance suggestive of the possibility of epilepsy of central origin.

Case 5

Summary. Female aged 11 years. Toxaemic pregnancy, poor balance and tendency to drop objects with resulting temper tantrums. Thought to be lazy and stupid. Crossed dominance, untidy handwriting, defective right–left orientation. WISC Verbal IQ 114, Performance IQ 92, Reading Quotient 108. EEG epileptogenic disturbances of central origin.

Report. A.C., the elder of two sisters, was born at term after a normal labour and delivery. Her mother was treated by bed rest at home for toxaemia which was present in the latter 6 weeks of pregnancy. Her early development seemed normal, but when she first went to school her parents realised that she was more inclined to lose her balance and to drop objects from her hands than were other children. She had much greater difficulty than others in the performance of manual skills such as writing, drawing, knitting and sewing, and frustration over these difficulties often provoked temper tantrums. Her schoolteacher believed that the child was lazy and stupid.

At the time she was examined at the age of 11 years 2 months, she was still enuretic at night. She was poor at ball games and still had difficulty in fastening buttons. Previously on WISC testing her Verbal score was 114 and Performance score 92. She was right-handed for writing and cleaning her teeth but left-handed for throwing a ball and left-eyed and left-footed. Her Reading Quotient was 108 and her writing was a little untidy. Right–left orientation was slightly defective and she was slow and made many mistakes before copying a cube correctly with matchsticks. Her performance with the insertion of objects into appropriate slots was poor and she was very slow in tying her shoelaces. No further physical signs were elicited.

The EEG showed occasional sharp transients in the right temporal region and less frequently on the left side. There was a single outburst of high amplitude, generalised, irregular spike and wave activity, suggesting a centrencephalic epileptic disturbance.

Case 6

Summary. Male aged 10 years. Three and a half weeks premature, prolonged labour, slow milestones, slow speech with difficulty in chewing and swallowing. Constructional apraxia, aggressive behaviour and restless. Speech and reading difficulties. WISC Verbal IQ 104, Performance IQ 111, Reading Quotient 59. EEG immature with right anterior abnormality.

Report. D.C., an only child, was born after $36\frac{1}{2}$ weeks gestation by normal delivery after a prolonged labour. His birth weight was 2.5 kg but his neonatal condition was satisfactory. He sat unaided at 15 months and walked at 2 years. Speech commenced at the age of $4\frac{1}{2}$ years but he could not construct sentences until he was 6 years old. He also had difficulty in chewing food and in swallowing in the first few years of life. As an older child he had difficulty in playing with constructional toys and at school shunned the use of pencils and paintbrushes because of the frustration that might ensue. He found it unusually difficult to learn to read and write. His frustration led to an aggressive behaviour pattern which was particularly evident at school. He was unable to dress or undress himself until the age of 9 years and when seen at the age of 10 years 8 months he was still unable to tie bows, brush his hair, ride a bicycle or participate adequately in ball games.

On examination he proved to be extremely restless, but was alert and co-operative. He was right-handed, right-eyed and right-footed and his speech had a mildly explosive quality with some substitution of consonants, but there was no facial or lingual apraxia. Reading performance was very poor with frequent transposition of letters, e.g. 'its' for 'sit' and he laboriously verbalised each component letter before often incorrectly enunciating a word. The Reading Quotient was estimated at 59. His writing was extremely untidy with occasional reversals and inversions of letters and he was unable to copy a cube adequately either by drawing or construction with matches. No further signs were elicited on physical examination. His IQ scores at the age of 10 years were 104 Verbal and 111 Performance.

The EEG was unstable and immature with fronto-parietal bursts of suspiciously sharp alpha activity. Outbursts of paroxysmal and intermittent slow wave activity on hyperventilation were followed immediately afterwards with definite high voltage sharp waves in the right fronto-parietal region. The findings were those of immaturity together with some evidence suggesting a right anterior lesion.

Case 7

Summary. Male aged 12 years. Born by forceps delivery after prolonged labour. Delayed walking and difficulty with writing and drawing and thought to be educationally subnormal. Left-handed with crossed dominance. Developmental dysarthria, facial and lingual apraxia, simultagnosia, finger agnosia, astereognosis and poor tactile localisation. Ideational, ideomotor con-structional and dressing apraxia. Mild impairment of joint position sense in fingers and toes. WISC Verbal IQ 89, Performance IQ 53, Reading Quotient 102. EEG mild to moderate diffuse abnormality.

Report. I.M., the oldest of four children, was born by forceps delivery at term after a labour lasting $2\frac{1}{2}$ days. His neonatal condition was satisfactory but walking was delayed until the age of 2 years 2 months. He had always found it difficult to play with constructional toys and later to write and draw. When he was sent to school the school doctor felt that he was educationally subnormal despite the fact that he learned to read quite well.

On assessment at the age of $12\frac{1}{2}$ years he lacked insight into his difficulties and appeared rather apprehensive. He was barely able to hop and could only descend steps singly. He was left-handed (with a family history of left-handedness), but right-eyed and right-footed. His speech lacked normal fluency and he seemed to force his words out with occasional mispronunciation of consonants. There was an associated facial and lingual apraxia of moderate degree. His Reading Quotient was 102 but his writing and drawings were decidedly immature. There was slight difficulty in recognising the significance of simple pictures as a whole although details were well appreciated. Severe bilateral finger agnosia, mild astereognosis and poor tactile localisation were present. He exhibited an ideational and ideomotor apraxia as well as a marked constructional (Figure 3.1) and dressing apraxia. No defect could be found in the motor system but he made occasional errors in the testing of joint position sense in his fingers and toes. His Verbal score was 89 and Performance score 53 on the WISC.

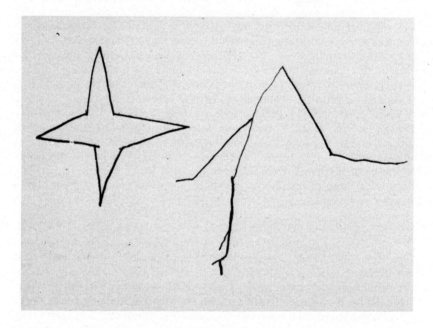

Figure 3.1. Case 7: Attempt to copy a star figure drawn by examiner (child aged $12\frac{1}{2}$ years). Reproduced with the kind permission of the editor of *Brain*.

The EEG was a low-voltage featureless record with some fast activity and poorly developed alpha. An excessive amount of low-voltage theta and delta was present and there was a general suppression of activity over the parietal regions even during hyperventilation. The appearances were those of a mild to moderate disturbance especially in both parietal regions.

Case 8

Summary. Male aged 11 years. Four and a half weeks premature, jaundiced at birth, delayed motor milestones. Frequent falls, ineptness at all physical tasks with aloofness, tenseness and agitation. Right–left orientation, finger agnosia, bilateral graphaesthesia. Apraxia of ideational, ideomotor, motor, constructional, and dressing types. Convergent squint. WISC Verbal IQ 109, Performance IQ 64, Reading Quotient 95. EEG diffusely abnormal and suspicion of right posterior lesion.

Report. P.B., the elder of two children, was born $4\frac{1}{2}$ weeks prematurely and had a birth weight of 2.7 kg. Apart from being jaundiced at birth his neonatal condition was good. Developmental motor milestones were somewhat delayed in that he sat up at 10 months and walked at 2 years. As a small child he had frequent falls and difficulty in getting up from the floor. Physical and manual performance were always retarded in such acts as unscrewing jars, opening doors and dressing. At the age of 8 years his teacher recognised that he was intelligent but commented that he could not do his handwork and was unsuccessful at gymnastics. Inability to play games with other children led to an aloofness and lack of confidence coupled with tenseness and agitation for which psychiatric treatment was sought.

When examined at the age of 11 years 4 months, he seemed unduly forthright in his manner and lacked insight into his considerable disabilities. He was right-handed, right-eyed and right-footed and the Reading Quotient was 95. Right–left orientation and finger sense were mildly impaired and bilateral graphaesthesia was present. He had no idea of how to fold a sheet of notepaper for insertion into an envelope and when asked to salute, touched the back of his head. A moderate degree of constructional, dressing and motor apraxia was present. There was a slight convergent squint due to weakness of abduction of the right eye, but this had been present since he had measles at the age of 2 years; otherwise no further neurological signs were elicited. WISC scores were 109 Verbal and 64 Performance.

The EEG showed a considerable excess of slow activity over both hemispheres posteriorly. On the left side there was an abolition of alpha rhythm posteriorly with early slowing on hyperventilation and lack of driving with photic stimulation. The findings were those of a diffuse abnormality with considerable suspicion of a left posterior lesion.

Case 9

Summary. Female aged 9 years. Face presentation. Older twin sister died from birth trauma. Frequently dropped objects out of hands. Awkward manually. Operation for squint age 5 years. Sinistral, developmental dysarthria. Topographical and finger agnosia. Moderate constructional and dressing apraxia. WISC Verbal IQ 94, Performance IQ 72, Reading Quotient 80. EEG moderate diffuse abnormality.

Report. L.T., the younger twin of a first pregnancy, was delivered as a face presentation. Her twin sister died at the age of 3 days from cerebral haemorrhage due to presumed birth trauma. She walked and talked at a normal age but was unsteady on her legs and frequently dropped objects out of her hands. She was always awkward manually and had great difficulty in learning to write. At 5 years she had an operation on both eyes for squint.

When seen at the age of 9 years 8 months she was rather slow in her movements and responses. She was left-handed, left-eyed and left-footed and there was a strong family history of left-handedness. Her speech was slow and clipped with defective formulation of consonants. The Reading Quotient was 80 and her writing to dictation was very slow with many spelling errors and incorrect letter construction with reversals. Her drawing of a clockface showed some disturbance of appreciation of extrapersonal space and a reversed figure 9 (Figure 3.2). She had mild finger agnosia, but moderate constructional and dressing apraxia. Further neurological examination was essentially negative. The WISC Verbal score was 94 and Performance 72.

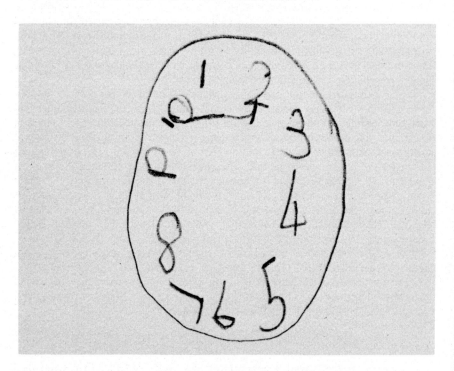

Figure 3.2. Case 9: Attempt to draw a clock-face and insert hands at 10 to 2 (child aged 9¾ years). Reproduced with the kind permission of the editor of *Brain*.

The EEG showed a dominant delta posterior rhythm in an extremely polyrhythmic record suggesting moderate diffuse abnormality.

Case 10

Summary. Male aged 9 years. Prolonged labour, slow development, thought to be lazy. Retarded reading and writing. Ambidextrous, right–left disorientation, finger agnosia, constructional apraxia. EEG left-occipital spike focus.

Report. G.G., the second of four children, was delivered normally after a prolonged labour. His early development was a little retarded and he had greater difficulty than his schoolmates in fastening buttons and shoelaces and was generally clumsy in his manual performance. His headmistress at first regarded him as being lazy because he would not attempt to write or draw. His parents and three siblings were left-handed and he himself was ambidextrous, left-eyed and right-footed.

On examination at the age of 9 years 5 months, he spoke with a heavy lisp. He could read only two words of Schonell's reading test R1 ('egg' and 'sit') and misread 'bun' for 'tea' and 'book' for 'frog'. He had complete right–left disorientation and severe finger agnosia. There were numerous inversions and spelling mistakes in his writing (Figure 3.3) and in addition he had a marked

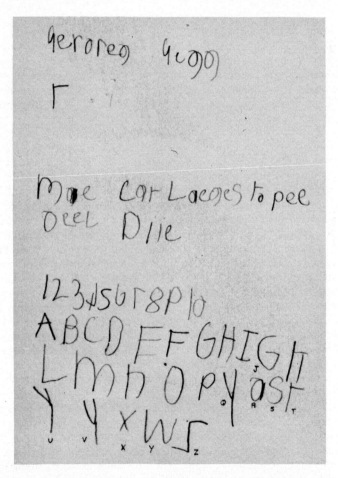

Figure 3.3. Case 10: Writing to dictation 'George Gregg: 7: my cat likes to play all day'. Below is attempt at writing figures 1 to 10 and the alphabet (child aged 9½ years). Reproduced with the kind permission of the editor of *Brain*.

constructional apraxia. Although no signs were elicited on neurological examination, the EEG recordist observed occasional twitching movements of his right thumb which were synchronous with a left occipital spike focus. His WISC scores were Verbal 82 and Performance 64.

The EEG was generally unstable and asymmetrical with excessively slow left-sided activity and a well-marked left occipital spike focus. There were brief bilateral outbursts of polyspike and irregular slow wave discharges which were generalised, synchronous and more or less symmetrical. The appearances suggested the presence of a centrencephalic seizure disorder with a left posterior focal epileptogenic lesion.

Case 11

Summary. Male aged 11 years. Delayed walking, improper articulation, dribbling with defective chewing and swallowing. Occasional grand mal. Ambidextrous, untidy, right–left disorientation, right sensory inattention, finger agnosia, astereognosis, impaired two-point discrimination and joint position sense, graphaesthesia, constructional apraxia. Choreiform movements in tongue and limbs (? pseudoathetosis). WISC Verbal IQ 99, Performance IQ 83, Reading Quotient 98. EEG normal.

Report. C.W. was the younger of two children. His perinatal history was normal but he first began to walk at 21 months. Although speech was not delayed, it was indistinct and he had a prolonged tendency to omit the ends of words. Even as an older child he dribbled frequently from the mouth and had some difficulty with chewing and swallowing. Between the ages of 9 and 10 years he sustained three attacks of loss of consciousness which were regarded as epileptic in origin and for which he was receiving phenobarbitone 30 mg b.d. Until the time of examination all physical activities were clumsily executed.

At the age of 11 years 3 months he was found to be ambidextrous, right-eyed and right-footed. When speaking he occasionally left off the ends of words and mispronounced several consonants. His writing and drawing was slow, deliberate and untidy, but his reading was adequate, with a Reading Quotient of 98. There was a mild right–left disorientation and on simultaneous bilateral cutaneous stimulation he occasionally missed the right-sided stimulus. He had finger agnosia of moderate degree and was unable to identify objects that were placed in his hands by tactile sensation alone. The threshold to two-point discrimination was increased to greater than 4 cm on all his fingers and 6 cm on the soles of both feet.

Joint position sense was grossly abnormal in all fingers and toes, but light touch, vibration, pain and temperature sense were all intact. Bilateral graphaesthesia was present. He had a moderate constructional apraxia. Abnormal movements of choreiform nature were present in the tongue, both upper limbs and the left lower limb. They were slightly more pronounced with eyes closed than open and were considered to be pseudoathetotic. WISC testing revealed a Verbal score of 99 and a Performance score of 83.

The EEG was within normal limits.

Case 12

Summary. Male aged 9 years. Delayed speech, untidy writing, ambidextrous, developmental dysarthria. Right–left disorientation, finger agnosia, constructional and dressing apraxia. Squint, choreiform movements. WISC Verbal IQ 77, Performance IQ 104. EEG mild to moderate abnormality with suspicion of left posterior temporal lesion.

Report. A.D., the second of a family of four children, had a normal perinatal history. Early physical development was normal, but acquisition of speech was very delayed in that he was only capable of using adequate sentences at the age of 5 or 6 years. His writing was always untidy and he had difficulty with dressing, but otherwise could use his hands quite well with toys, 'meccano', plasticine and drawing.

At the age of 9 years 8 months he was examined and found to be ambidextrous, right-eyed and right-footed. His speech was poorly articulated; parts of words were omitted and he made some substitutions in the pronunciation of consonants. Words were enunciated slowly and deliberately, and he was slow in the comprehension and execution of simple commands. His writing too was slow and untidy with unusual substitutions of letters and the tendency to omit the ends of words (Figure 3.4). There was some right–left disorientation and finger agnosia, and a mild constructional and dressing apraxia. A bilateral external rectus weakness was present with Duane's syndrome on the right side. The only other abnormal finding in the nervous system was the presence of mild choreiform movements of both hands, fingers and toes. The WISC gave a Verbal score of 77 and Performance score of 104.

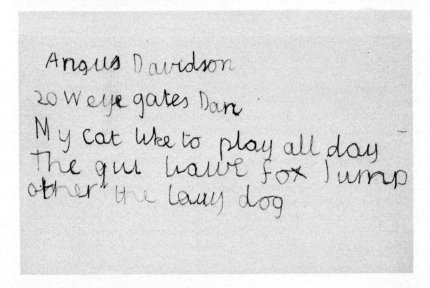

Figure 3.4. Case 12: Writing to dictation 'Angus Davidson 20 Waygate Drive. My cat likes to play all day. The quick brown fox jumps over the lazy dog' (child aged $9\frac{3}{4}$ years). Reproduced with the kind permission of the editor of *Brain*.

The EEG was unstable and showed excessive theta and delta activity posteriorly with one or two generalised paroxysms of slow waves. At times more slow activity was present on the left side posteriorly than the right. The appearances were those of a moderate degree of instability giving rise to generalised mild to moderate abnormality and some slight suspicion of the presence of a left posterior temporal lesion.

Case 13

Summary. Female aged 12 years. Forceps delivery, face presentation. Delayed walking and speech and very delayed physical skills. Stiff awkward gait, restless, writing difficulty, right–left orientation, finger agnosia and graphaesthesia. Ideomotor, motor, constructional and dressing apraxias. Slow tongue movements and choreiform movements. Mild impairment joint position sense. WISC Verbal IQ 85, Performance IQ 44. EEG mild non-specific abnormality.

Report. M.M., an only child, was delivered with forceps as a face presenta-tion. Oedema and bruising of the face did not subside for a month after delivery. She sat up at 9 months, walked at 22 months and did not speak in sentences until the age of 3 years. She was always severely handicapped by an inability to use her hands adequately and was unable to drink unaided from a cup until 3 years, brush her teeth until 9 years and open doors or skip until 10 years of age. At the time of her most recent medical examination at the age of 12 years 7 months she had still not managed to dress or undress or brush her hair by herself and had never been able to ride a tricycle or bicycle. Her gait was stiff and awkward and she hopped on either foot with great deliberation. She was restless throughout the examination but concentration and co-operation were good. Her handwriting was slow and there was poor alignment and formulation of letters with several spelling errors. There seemed particular difficulty in holding the pencil. Profound right–left disorientation and finger agnosia were present together with bilateral graphaesthesia. Ideomotor and motor apraxia and severe constructional and dressing apraxia were demonstrated. She had slow movements of her tongue and difficulty in copying lingual and labial movements. Slight choreiform movements of the tongue, face, neck and all four limbs were observed. The deep tendon reflexes and both plantar responses were normal. She made occasional errors in testing joint position sense in the toes, but other modalities of sensation were normal. WISC testing revealed a Verbal score of 85 and a Performance score of 44.

The EEG showed persistent eye and muscle artifact but with well-developed posterior alpha rhythm and some diffuse excess of theta and delta over the vertex and temporal regions. The appearances were those of a mild, non-specific abnormality without clear evidence of any focal cerebral lesion.

Case 14

Summary. Male aged 14 years. Disturbed social background. Delayed respirations after delivery. Restless, fidgety, lack of concentration, defective handwriting, outbursts of temper. Reading and writing difficulties. Right–left disorientation and finger agnosia. Generalised hypotonia, dressing apraxia, choreiform movements. WISC Verbal IQ 85, Performance IQ 94, Reading Quotient 45. EEG mild to moderate non-specific abnormality.

Report. G.F. came from a disturbed social background, and was the youngest of three siblings. Respirations were delayed for several minutes after delivery. He became restless and fidgety during his fourth year and this was thought to have followed an attack of 'Saint Vitus' Dance'. When he first went to school he lacked concentration and was so very unsteady with his hands that writing and drawing were extremely defective. Generally his behaviour was good, but occasionally there were outbursts of temper. He was right-handed, right-eyed and right-footed.

At the age of 14 years 3 months his Reading Quotient was only 45 and he frequently confused letters which were inversions or reversals of one another such as 'd', 'b' and 'p'. There was complete right–left disorientation and mild finger agnosia. His writing was barely recognisable as such because of poor formulation of letters and numerous spelling errors. His movements were all slow and clumsy and resulted in untidy drawings. He had a mild dressing apraxia. There was some generalised hypotonia and he exhibited mild choreiform movements of his tongue and all four limbs. On the WISC his Verbal score was 85 and Performance score 94.

The EEG showed excessive theta activity and even delta discharges. There was a well-developed, symmetrical alpha rhythm posteriorly and the appearances suggested mild to moderate non-specific abnormality with no clear evidence of a focal cerebral lesion.

Group II

Case 15

Summary. Male aged 8 years. Mother with congenital left hemiparesis. Normal development until febrile illness aged 15 months, followed by speech retardation. Clumsy gait, difficulty with dressing, untidy with eating. Poor mixer with frequent tantrums and recent improvement. Constructional and dressing apraxia. Developmental dysarthria. Right–left disorientation, finger agnosia and choreiform movements. WISC Verbal IQ 135, Performance IQ 108, Reading Quotient 121. EEG asymmetrical with left parietal delta suggesting a left-sided cerebral lesion.

Report. M.J., the elder of two brothers and the son of a clergyman, was delivered in a motor vehicle by his father, but otherwise the perinatal history was unremarkable. His mother, an intelligent woman, was minimally incapacitated by a congenital left hemiparesis and was herself delivered with forceps. He walked unaided at 13 months and had a vocabulary of about 20 words by the age of 1 year. At 15 months he had a febrile illness with drowsiness for 2 or 3 days and recovered spontaneously, but after this time sensible speech was lost. At 2 years his vocabulary was confined to a few words and he was unable to speak in sentences until aged $3\frac{1}{2}$ years. The speech that he re-acquired was quite normal. As he grew older it became obvious that his gait was clumsy and he was slow in learning acts such as dressing and undressing. Even then he was liable to put his clothes on back to front. He was always untidy in eating habits and in all manual activities. He did not mix well with other children and from the age of 3 years had frequent tantrums. There had been a considerable improvement in all his disabilities in the previous few years. On examination at the age of 8 years 2 months he had a moderate constructional and dressing apraxia, but no further signs and it was felt that these might be the neurological sequelae of an encephalitic illness occurring at 15 months of age. On the WISC his Verbal score was 135 and Performance score 108.

The EEG was asymmetrical and showed excessive slow activity mainly in delta frequency range in the left parietal region and further activated by hyperventilation. The appearances led to suspicion of the presence of a left-sided cerebral lesion.

Case 16

Summary. Male aged 13 years. Severe whooping cough at 3 months and pneumonia at 12 months and 15 months with subsequent recurrent bronchitis. Delayed motor development and excessively clumsy with topographical agnosia. Handwriting difficulty and disturbed body image. Ungainly gait, simultagnosia, right–left confusion and finger agnosia. Motor, constructional and facial apraxia with dribbling. Fidgety, restless, pseudoathetosis, astereognosis and graphaesthesia. Equivocal left plantar. WISC Verbal IQ 80, Performance IQ 62, Reading Quotient 62. EEG mild to moderate abnormality with suspicion of left-sided lesion.

Report. J.B., the younger of two children, thrived until the age of 3 months when he had a severe attack of whooping cough. At 12 months he had pneumonia and was nursed in hospital in an oxygen tent for a week. There was a second attack of pneumonia at 15 months followed by recurrent winter bronchitis until he was aged 7 years.

Motor development was delayed; he sat at 15 months and walked at 3 years, but speech developed normally. He was always a clumsy child and when he started school at 5 years was so awkward and his topographical sense so poor that his schoolteacher had to detail two other boys to take him up and down stairs and along passages. At 8 years he was unable to read and doing badly at school. He could not hop or jump and could not copy drawings, letters or figures.

When tested on the WISC he had a Verbal score of 87 and Performance score of 44. Handwriting was crude, showing many reversals and his drawing extremely poor. His principal difficulty seemed to be in relating the different parts of his body to one another.

When reviewed at the age of 13 years 8 months he was found to walk and run in a very ungainly fashion. He was unable to hop on either foot or to jump, although muscular power was normal. He was right-handed and right-footed. Speech was normal, but he made numerous errors with reading for although he could read parts of words correctly he was mostly unable to recognise the words as a whole. The Reading Quotient was 62. Similarly when interpreting simple pictures he could usually recognise individual detail, but was unable to appreciate the picture as a whole. His handwriting was untidy and several words and letters were unrecognisable. He had a mild right–left confusion, but a severe finger agnosia, motor apraxia and constructional apraxia (Figure 3.5).

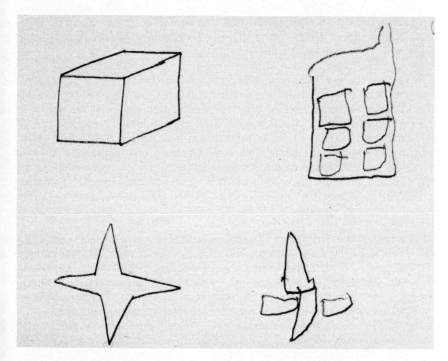

Figure 3.5. Case 16: Attempt to copy a cube and a star figure drawn by examiner (child aged 13¾ years). Reproduced with the kind permission of the editor of *Brain*.

There was an apraxia for facial movements and he constantly dribbled from both corners of his mouth. He was extremely fidgety and restless, but exhibited as well a pseudoathetosis of the outstretched hands. In contrast to an examination at the age of 9 years his two-point discrimination was normal, joint position sense was only mildly impaired and ability to recognise objects placed in his hands was only moderately impaired although graphaesthesia was profound. On this occasion the left plantar response was equivocal, whereas before it was regarded as flexor. A further assessment on WISC testing had placed the Verbal score at 80 and Performance score at 62.

The EEG was rather unstable and asymmetrical with more slow activity on the left side than on the right and some suppression of left anterior beta activity as compared with the right. Hyperventilation produced some left-sided sharp activity. The changes were those of a mild to moderate non-specific disturbance with some suspicion of a left-sided lesion.

Case 17

Summary. Male aged 17 years. Congenital right cataract removed at age 7 years with subsequent blindness in that eye. Clumsy motor activities including dressing and undressing. Pathologically brisk tendon jerks and bilateral extensor plantar responses. Right—left disorientation, finger agnosia, constructional apraxia. WISC Verbal IQ 82, Performance IQ 54, Reading age $12\frac{1}{2}$ years. EEG non-focal epileptiform activity.

Report. S.N., the oldest of three siblings, was born with a right-sided cataract which was submitted to operation at 7 years, but iritis and subsequent blindness developed in the eye. When he first started school at the age of 5 years it became evident that he was clumsier than his peers. Later he showed particular ineptitude in the use of tools and in handwriting and he had much difficulty in learning to climb and skip. Dressing and undressing always presented a problem and he did not learn to brush his hair adequately or to ride a bicycle until the age of 14 years. When examined at 14 years 10 months he was found to have pathologically brisk tendon jerks and bilateral extensor plantar responses. On the WISC his Verbal score was 82 and Performance score 54.

On assessment at the age of 17 years 4 months, he was a tall shy youth who was right-handed and right-footed. His speech was adequate, but his reading age was only $12\frac{1}{2}$ years and writing was very untidy with defective formation of words and letters. There was mild right—left disorientation and finger agnosia with a moderate degree of constructional apraxia. Further physical examination confirmed the presence of a minimal spastic quadriparesis.

The EEG showed a predominance of theta and delta activity posteriorly which was of lower voltage on the left side. Sharp activity together with several paroxysms of polyspikes and slow waves were present in the right anterior regions. The appearances suggested epileptiform discharges of central origin and the possibility of a right frontal lesion.

Case 18

Summary. Female aged 13 years. Surgical induction for antepartum haemorrhage. Delayed walking, poor concentration, mislaying objects, losing herself easily and untidy motor activity. Occasional blank spells and diurnal incontinence. Right—left disorientation, topographical agnosia, constructional apraxia, convergent squint, static hand tremor, impaired fine movements of left hand and possible left hyperreflexia. WISC Verbal IQ 97, Performance IQ 82, Reading Quotient 110. EEG suggested a right-sided posterior lesion.

Report. D.S., the second child of a family of four children, was delivered normally at 38 weeks' gestation following a surgical induction for mild antepartum haemorrhage. Walking was delayed until the age of 2 years although speech was acquired at the normal time. She always lacked concentration, frequently mislaid objects and got lost easily. Schoolwork was below standard at the outset and she was unable to cope with sewing or knitting. Writing and constructive tasks such as making her bed were very untidy. Inversions in her handwriting were frequent until the age of 9 years. She was clumsy in her manipulations of buttons and shoelaces and was unable to ride a tricycle until she was aged 6 years.

Her parents for some time had noticed her having occasional 'absences' when her eyes would become 'blank' and she would remain mentally inaccessible for a few seconds. She also suffered from diurnal incontinence although it was not established whether the incontinence was associated with the 'absences'.

She was examined at $13\frac{1}{2}$ years and found to be right-handed, right-eyed and right-footed with some right—left disorientation and topographical agnosia. Her Reading Quotient was 110 and writing was unremarkable. A moderate finger agnosia was present and despite many attempts she was unable to copy a cube design from matchsticks.

Further examination revealed a convergent squint due to right lateral rectus weakness and there was a fine static tremor of both hands. Fine finger movements of the left hand were impaired and the deep tendon reflexes were possibly slightly brisker on the left side although both plantars were flexor. WISC scores were 97 Verbal and 82 Performance.

The EEG tracing was asymmetrical where activity over the left cerebral hemisphere appeared normal, but on the right side posteriorly there was a considerable excess of delta activity which was often irregular. Initial striking asymmetry with more slow activity developing on the right side than on the left was noted with hyperventilation. The appearances suggested the presence of a posterior right-sided lesion.

Case 19

Summary. Female aged 9 years. Rather low birth weight, delayed respirations, neonatal jaundice with history of Rh incompatibility. Severe febrile convulsive illness at the age of 2 months and unable to walk or speak until aged 3 years. Slow motor development and thought to be educationally retarded. Unable to read, sinistral, disturbed topographical sense and simultagnosia. Finger agnosia, constructional and dressing apraxia. WISC Verbal IQ 81, Performance IQ 44 and Reading Quotient approximately 50. EEG moderately severe diffuse abnormality.

Report. M.S. was the second of three children. The fourth pregnancy ended in stillbirth at $7\frac{1}{2}$ months gestation through Rhesus incompatibility. The patient was delivered normally after a 9-month gestation period, but her birth weight was only 2.3 kg, and oxygen was administered for 15 minutes because of some delay in the onset of respiration. Although jaundiced for the first week of life, transfusion was considered unnecessary. At the age of 2 months she was seriously ill with fever and convulsions and admitted to a hospital in

Glasgow where the diagnosis of meningitis was considered, but not confirmed by the time of apparent full recovery. She was unable to walk unaided or utter single words until aged 3 years, and only learned to drink without assistance from a cup at $3\frac{1}{2}$ years. At the age of 5 years she first managed to ride her tricycle, brush her teeth and negotiate doorknobs and doorhandles. At school she was considered to be educationally retarded and at the age of $9\frac{1}{2}$ years was barely able to read or write. She was left-handed.

On examination she could read correctly only three words of Schonell's test R 1 and read 'shop' for 'school', 'dog' for 'bun' and 'sheet' for 'sit'. Her writing was extremely untidy; she was unable to write her name correctly and many letters were curiously constructed. Drawings of a clock-face (Figure 3.6) and house revealed a disturbance of topographical sense. She had difficulty in under-

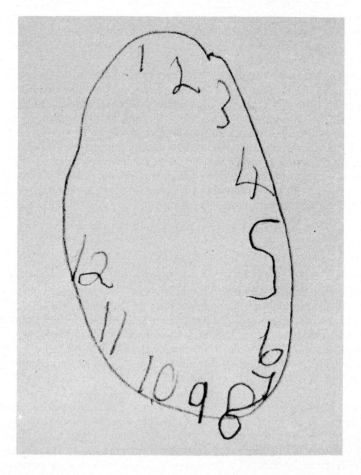

Figure 3.6. Case 19: Attempt to draw a clock-face showing inability to insert the hands at 10 to 2 (child aged $9\frac{1}{2}$ years). Reproduced with the kind permission of the editor of *Brain*.

standing the meaning of simple pictures although details were well appreciated and finger sense was grossly impaired. A constructional apraxia (Figure 3.7) and mild dressing apraxia were evident. On the WISC her Verbal score was 81 and Performance 44.

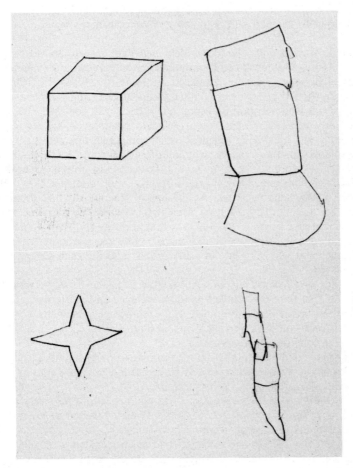

Figure 3.7. Case 19: Attempt to copy a cube and star figure drawn by examiner (child aged $9\frac{1}{2}$ years). Reproduced with the kind permission of the editor of *Brain*.

The EEG was a low-voltage record with a fleeting appearance of alpha rhythms posteriorly and showing dominant mixed theta and delta discharges. There was delayed recovery to baseline activity after the resumption of normal respirations. The appearances were those of a moderately severe diffuse abnormality with no definite focal changes.

Case 20

Summary. Female aged 17 years. Forceps delivery, prolonged labour with cephalhaematoma. Neonatal jaundice, requiring transfusion and delayed milestones. Right-sided Jacksonian seizures with occasional convulsion. Squint, clumsy motor activity, sinistral, finger agnosia, constructional apraxia and pathologically brisk deep reflexes. WISC Verbal IQ 90, Performance IQ 77. EEG sharp activity bilaterally with excessive instability on hyperventilation. Previous EEGs had shown much epileptiform activity.

Report. D.W., an only child, was delivered with forceps following labour lasting 72 hours, and developed a cephalhaematoma a few hours later. Within 24 hours of birth she became jaundiced and was transfused. For the first 2 weeks of life she fed poorly and vomited frequently. Sitting was delayed until 20 months and walking until $3\frac{1}{4}$ years, but speech was acquired at a normal time. Between the ages of 5 and 9 years she had experienced, at approximately monthly intervals, Jacksonian seizures which sometimes affected the right arm and mouth and sometimes the left arm and thumb. The attacks generally lasted for only a few seconds at a time, but occasionally would proceed to a generalised convulsion. They were currently well controlled by regular medication with phenobarbitone. At the age of 9 years she had a corrective operation for squint that had been present from birth. By the time that she went to school at 5 years it was obvious that she was clumsy with her hands and had difficulty in using pencil and crayons. She was particularly maladroit at ball games and was very late in using a knife and fork and getting dressed and undressed.

At the age of 17 years she was still unable to fasten her shoelaces. When examined at that time she was left-handed, left-eyed and left-footed and it was noted that her father was left-handed. Her reading age was at the 12-year-old level and writing was a little shaky and untidy. She had a right-sided finger agnosia and constructional apraxia.

On physical examination, all deep tendon reflexes were pathologically brisk, but both plantar responses were flexor. Sensation was normal. WISC IQ scores were 90 Verbal and 77 Performance.

The EEG showed a mild excess of theta activity with a few isolated sharp transients over both hemispheres. Hyperventilation resulted in excessive and paroxysmal breakdown with asymmetry comprising slower activity on the right than on the left. Previous EEGs had shown evidence of severe focal abnormalities over the right hemisphere with outbursts of slow waves, spikes and sharp waves.

Case 21

Summary. Female aged 14 years. Tuberculous meningitis aged 2 years, followed by prolonged blindness. Further development very delayed with unsteady gait and manual activity. Constructional apraxia, motor apraxia and topographical agnosia; hyperreflexia and extensor plantars. WISC Verbal IQ 95, Performance IQ 44, Reading Quotient 101. EEG left posterior lesion.

Report. P.P. had progressed normally until she developed tuberculous arthritis of the left knee at 18 months and tuberculous meningitis the following year. At the onset of the meningitis she was unconscious for several days and during the course of that illness lost her vision completely for a period of 15 months, but eventually it was fully restored. She did not relearn to walk confidently until the age of 6 or 7 years and she was still clumsy on her legs and with her hands. She had a very labile and sensitive temperament.

At the age of 14 years 8 months, running, jumping and hopping were performed awkwardly and unsteadily. She was right-handed, left-eyed and right-footed. Speech was normal and her Reading Quotient was 101. She had a severe finger agnosia and a moderate degree of constructional apraxia and motor apraxia and lack of topographical sense. Her visual acuity was normal and there was no optic atrophy, but a small patch of healed choroiditis was present below the left optic disc. Tone and deep tendon reflexes were increased in the lower limbs and both plantar responses were extensor. A slight action tremor was observed in the left upper limb. Her Verbal IQ was 95 and Performance IQ 44 on the WISC.

The EEG showed a slight excess of theta activity over the right hemisphere, but the left side was dominated by delta discharges. Sometimes these were irregular and sometimes rhythmical especially posteriorly. There was an initial exaggeration of the asymmetry during hyperventilation followed by the sudden development of generalised, slow activity of mixed, irregular, rhythmical type. Recruitment with photic stimulation was much better developed over the right hemisphere than the left. The appearances strongly suggested the presence of a posterior left-sided lesion with a general disturbance of function over most of the left hemisphere.

RESULTS

Detailed analysis of the findings in the children of Groups I and II is provided in Table 3.3. Additional information not given in the table is discussed here. Firstly, it should be mentioned that there was no family history of clumsiness, but the mother of one of the children in Group II had a mild congenital hemiparesis. In no case did the maternal age at the time of the child's birth exceed 36 years. A behaviour disorder was present to some extent in most of the cases. Ocular dominance was disregarded in the assessment of crossed lateralities as Jasper and Raney (1937), confirmed by McFie (1952), found no correspondence between hemisphere dominance and preference for one eye, nor between eyedness and handedness.

In nine children of Group I there was some degree of abnormal articulation and four of these had an associated facial and lingual apraxia. These articulation defects, according to the classification devised by Morley, Court and Miller (1954), were all to be regarded as forms of developmental dysarthria. In each of the five cases with developmental dysarthria in which abnormal movements of the lips, tongue and palate were not demonstrated, the defect was considered to be an articulatory apraxia. The latter is presumed to be due to a disturbance of function arising at a higher level in the effector

Table 3.3. Analysis of cases of Group I (isolated apraxia and agnosia) and Group II (apraxia and agnosia with minimal neurological signs)

Specific observations at latest examination	Group I (14 cases)	Group II (7 cases)
Average age	11 years 10 months	14 years 3 months
Males	10	3
Females	4	4
Abnormal perinatal factors[a]	10	3
Incidence of firstborn	8	4
Delayed walking (beyond 2 years)	4	4
Completely or principally left-handed	6	3
Crossed laterality	6	1
Alexia	4	2
Agraphia (apraxic or agnosic)	13	7
Articulation defect without lingual apraxia	5	1
Articulation defect with lingual apraxia	4	1
'Acalculia' (see text)	4	1
Right–left disorientation	10	4
Finger agnosia	10	5
Topographical agnosia	3	3
Ideational apraxia	4	1
Ideomotor apraxia	5	2
Motor apraxia	6	2
Constructional apraxia	11	6
Dressing apraxia	13	7
'Choreiform movements'	4	1
'Cortical' sensory loss	3	1
Higher WISC Verbal score	11	7
Incidence of squint	3	2
Incidence of epilepsy	2	2

[a] Includes one or more of the following: pre-eclampsia, eclampsia, prolonged labour, prematurity, abnormal delivery, severe jaundice.
Reproduced with the kind permission of the editor of *Brain*.

pathways of speech in the nervous system than in a patient with facial and lingual apraxia.

Poor writing, which was almost universal, was probably largely a function of an associated constructional apraxia (apraxic agraphia), but when it was also associated with alexia it was regarded as mainly a function of the latter. At least five of the children had significantly low arithmetic subscores in proportion to their overall Verbal score on the WISC and obviously they had a further specific inability to calculate (acalculia). A less obvious specific calculation defect was present in other children, but it was not possible to determine the exact number because of the continuous range between subnormal and above normal ability to calculate. All but three of the children had higher Verbal than Performance IQ scores and in the group as a whole this disparity is statistically significant ($P < 0.01$, Table 3.4).

There was generally a close correlation between the co-existence of ideational, ideomotor and motor apraxia in any one individual. Either a constructional or a dressing apraxia was observed in every instance and most children had both.

Table 3.4. Most recent IQ values

Case	Verbal IQ	Performance IQ	Excess of verbal IQ
Group I			
1	116	93	23
2	120	106	14
3	95	78	17
4	104	71	33
5	114	92	22
6	104	111	−7
7	89	53	36
8	109	64	45
9	94	72	22
10	82	64	18
11	99	83	16
12	77	104	−27
13	85	44	41
14	85	94	−9
Group II			
15	135	108	27
16	80	62	18
17	82	54	28
18	97	82	15
19	81	44	37
20	90	77	13
21	95	44	51

The overall excess of Verbal over Performance IQ is statistically significant ($P < 0.01$). Reproduced with the kind permission of the editor of *Brain*.

It is of great interest that most of the children were restless and fidgety during the examination; four of them in Group I also exhibited abnormal movements, resembling those of chorea, and affecting their limbs and often the facial and lingual muscles. The significance of these choreiform movements is discussed below.

FOLLOW-UP INFORMATION

Cases 1, 2, 3 and 16 of this series were originally reported by Walton, Ellis and Court (1962). Their fifth case was not available for reassessment. Nearly six years after the last reported assessment, C.H. (1) and D.L. (2) had shown considerable spontaneous improvement. Both had continued to attend normal schools where they were regarded as average pupils. Both had WISC Verbal scores which were above average, and this might have explained their ability to learn to overcome their motor disabilities as they grew older.

On the other hand, D.N. (3) and J.B. (16), who were reassessed approximately five years later and who were less intelligent, were less able to learn to overcome their disabilities; however, the intensive special training and education which they had received throughout the period had helped them to compensate for their disabilities, and had lessened their behaviour disorder.

In all other cases the parents had noted that as the children grew older their disabilities had been less obvious. This improvement was so marked in Cases 5 and 15 that it seemed likely to be the result either of a regression of an underlying pathological process or of the acquisition of new patterns of neurophysiological activity concerned with learning and execution. It is admitted that valid scientific inferences from the results of follow-up information could only have been made adequately if specially devised tests of praxis and gnosis, standardised for age, had been applied to these children. At the time of this study there were no satisfactory methods in existence for making such assessments. In the following chapters, the development of such standardised tests is described.

ELECTROENCEPHALOGRAPHIC FINDINGS

A summary of the electroencephalographic findings is provided in Table 3.5. It will be observed that the degrees and types of abnormalities encountered were roughly of the same incidence in Groups I and II with the exception of major asymmetry which was more frequently seen in Group II. All but one of the 14 subjects in Group I with isolated apraxia and agnosia had an abnormal EEG. Eight subjects had moderate abnormalities and the remaining five were designated as mildly abnormal. In Group II where apraxia and agnosia occurred in association with other evidence of neurological dysfunction, all seven subjects had abnormal EEGs, five of which were moderately and two mildly abnormal. Fifteen of the children had diffuse abnormalities, most of which were mild, and seven exhibited background asymmetries which were usually of major significance. Apart from those children with asymmetries in the electroencephalograms there were six who had focal abnormalities. Although a history of epilepsy was forthcoming in only two subjects, seven of the EEGs exhibited epileptiform changes.

DISCUSSION

With few exceptions (sex incidence, crossed laterality, dysarthria and choreiform movements) the incidence of the various specific abnormalities was similar in Groups I and II. The cases of Group II should be regarded as having basically a form of minimal 'cerebral palsy' in addition to cognitive and executive defects of the type described. The clinical overlap between these two groups of cases might be used to support the contention that Group I is a collection of children with cerebral dysfunction who lie within the 'spectrum' of cerebral palsy. The high incidence of predisposing factors to anoxic birth injury seen in the group (prematurity, forceps delivery, etc.) as well as the presence of epilepsy and squint in some of the cases reinforces this argument as these factors are also accepted features in many children with established cerebral palsy. Benton (1973) advocates "study of the motor performances of MBD (minimal brain dysfunction) children with the aim of determining

Table 3.5. Summary of electroencephalographic data

Case	Mild diffuse disturbance	Marked diffuse disturbance	Minor asymmetry	Major asymmetry	Focal abnormality	Epileptiform discharges	Degree of abnormality
Group I							
1	+	−	+	−	−	−	Mild
2	+	−	−	−	+	−	Marked
3	−	−	−	−	+	+	Marked
4	+	+	−	−	−	+	Marked
5	+	−	−	−	−	+	Marked
6	−	+	−	−	+	−	Marked
7	+	−	−	−	−	−	Marked
8	+	−	−	+	−	−	Marked
9	−	−	−	−	−	−	Mild
10	+	−	−	−	+	+	Marked
11	+	−	−	−	−	−	Normal
12	−	−	+	−	−	−	Mild
13	+	−	−	−	−	−	Mild
14	+	−	−	−	−	−	Mild
Group II							
15	−	−	−	+	−	−	Marked
16	+	−	+	−	−	−	Mild
17	+	−	−	+	+	+	Marked
18	−	+	−	+	−	−	Marked
19	−	−	−	−	−	−	Mild
20	−	−	−	−	+	+	Marked
21	−	−	−	+	−	−	Marked

Reproduced with the kind permission of the editor of *Brain*.

whether some children do show apraxic defects that can be distinguished from more basic motor impairment . . .".

The follow-up information on the children in Group I also shows that spontaneous regressions of clumsiness and dysarthria can sometimes occur to a marked degree. This was particularly apparent in Case 2 and might be explained by the thesis that in some cases the condition is due to delayed maturation of part of the nervous system (*British Medical Journal*, 1962). Walton (1963) favoured the explanation that in some instances this clinical picture is the result of a defect of cerebral organisation in a neurophysiological rather than anatomical sense. This explanation obtains some support from the fact that in congenital dyslexia, a close clinical parallel, the disability does not arise from an acquired pathological lesion of any single area of the brain (Gallagher, 1960). McFie (1952) concluded from his studies of 12 cases of developmental dyslexia that the neurophysiological organisation corresponding to dominance had not been normally established. Zangwill (1960b) suggested that people with indeterminate cerebral dominance with regard to language and kindred processes are particularly vulnerable to the effects of stress such as minimal brain injury at birth; this may result in improper development of reading, writing, spatial judgement and directional control. There appears to be a rather direct relationship between the maturation of motor skills and the development of cerebral dominance (Benson and Geschwind, 1968). Drew (1956), in a study of three cases of familial dyslexia, discovered certain neurological findings believed to be comparable to abnormalities often seen in association with acquired 'word-blindness' due to involvement of the parietal lobes. Furthermore, in the Newcastle study, evidence for a structural rather than a physiological abnormality in the brain of a clumsy child was borne out by the high incidence of significant electroencephalographic changes.

It is possible that these children were a heterogenous group in which disordered cerebral anatomy (focal parietal lobe lesions resulting from injury) was the prime aetiological factor in some, whereas a fundamentally disordered physiology (perhaps defective establishment of physiological dominance) was the basis in the others. There was a singular lack of direct pathological evidence to confirm or refute either viewpoint since in none of the children under review was further neurological investigation warranted. In particular it was not felt that angiography or air encephalography was justified in any case. The fact that amelioration in the clinical state often occurred with time was of no special significance as this state of affairs does occur to some extent in some patients with 'cerebral palsy' in whom the disability is clearly the result of anatomical lesions. On the other hand the striking improvement which occurred in a few cases was more in favour of a process of physiological maturation and reorganisation.

Parallel studies and reports to the above, with emphasis on differing ranges of clinical manifestations, were given by Annell (1949), Benton (1959), Boshes and Myklebust (1964) and Paine (1962). Spillane (1942) and Critchley (1953) both have described instances of congenital Gerstmann's syndrome. Brain (1961) referred to the entity of developmental dyspraxia "which may be associated with developmental speech disorders and the subjects lack manual skills in general". Ford (1966) under the term 'Congenital Maladroitness' referred to children of normal intelligence who are slow to learn complex motor activities and suggests the possibility that this may be a specific developmental defect.

Anderson (1963), in a neurological appraisal of the hyperkinetic child, found minor neurological abnormalities in a high proportion of patients studied. He postulated that the entire syndrome was due to lack of adequate integration of various types of perceptual modalities as a result of minimal brain damage. This explanation might well have applied to many of the children in this series; however, it was felt that usually the disturbance of affect and of behaviour was a psychological reaction to the frustrations resulting from faulty manual skills in otherwise intelligent subjects. Ingram's (1963) suggested provisional classification of chronic brain syndromes in children other than the well-recognised entities of cerebral palsy, epilepsy and mental defect included 'Defined clinical syndromes with inconstant evidence of brain abnormality'. The examples cited in this category comprised specific retardation of speech development, specific developmental dyslexia and dysgraphia, and specific 'clumsiness'. These views are supported by the observations on the clumsy children reported in this section.

It has previously been suggested (Walton, Ellis and Court, 1962) that one of the salient features of the syndrome of developmental apraxia and agnosia is a marked discrepancy between Verbal and Performance scores on the Wechsler Intelligence Scale for Children and that the Verbal score is invariably the higher. This applied in all but three of the 21 cases (Cases 6, 12 and 14). Lower Verbal scores in these three children might have been explained by the fact that they all had relatively mild apraxia and agnosia, but also quite severe disorders of language. The same disparity of WISC IQ Scores has been confirmed in observations by Rutter, Tizard and Whitmore (1970) on clumsy children.

Critchley (1970) drew attention to cases of developmental dyslexia which were not always entirely 'pure' in the sense that the disability may not exist in complete isolation, but it may be combined with disorders of the body image, spatial perception, motor performance and of articulation. He alluded to relevant statements by Gooddy and Reinhold (1961) on right—left orientation and by Rabinovitch et al (1954) who were impressed by a non-specific clumsiness and awkwardness in motor function. If this suggestion is right, that aetiological factors are similar in the two groups, one would expect a considerable clinical overlap between subjects with developmental dyslexia on the one hand and children with developmental apraxia and agnosia on the other. It must, however, be noted that genetic evidence supplies a strong argument in favour of a constitutional and inherited cause for developmental dyslexia; but the more frequent lack of significant family history of similar difficulties in the clumsy children with or without dyslexia suggests that causal factors in the two groups possess important points of difference.

One of the remarkable features of the syndrome described is the practically universal 'fidgetiness' that was exhibited. Moreover, five of the children displayed at some time choreiform movements of varying degree. These movements, which tended to be accentuated by situations of emotional stress, were observed in muscles of the face, neck and limbs and to a lesser extent in the tongue. One EEG recordist observed independently that muscle and eye artifact was extremely frequent in the records because of twitching movements and restlessness in the children. Several other observers agreed independently that in none of these cases were the movements sufficiently severe to be classified as true choreo-athetosis; despite their superficial resemblance to the movements of chorea they were invariably abolished by voluntary effort, and could usually be controlled in the resting limbs by an effort of will; and there was rarely an associated hypotonia or reflex abnormality. Precisely the same observation has previously been noted by Prechtl and Stemmer (1962). These authors studied a group of children aged 9 and 12 years who had choreiform movements and who were originally referred because of behaviour disturbances at home or poor schoolwork. The children also had difficulties in reading and writing and in spatial perception and orientation. There was a high incidence of perinatal complications in this group of children and the authors suggested that the choreiform movements were the outcome of anoxic injury to the basal ganglia. It is tempting to ascribe the choreiform movements and the disturbances of praxis and gnosis to a common underlying lesion of the brain, but the fact that the movements were always bilateral makes this explanation improbable since widespread pathological change sufficient to give rise to such varied clinical manifestations would surely be expected to produce much more florid neurological findings, easily detectable on examination. An alternative suggestion is that these movements were a physiological function of underlying apraxia and/or agnosia and might be termed 'searching movements'.

The fact that an additional 17 'clumsy children' had been recognised and investigated since the initial report of Walton, Ellis and Court (1962) some two years previously, supported their contention that this syndrome was much commoner than was generally realised. Probably many such children were now attending ordinary schools and were being wrongly classified as lazy or backward or as suffering from behaviour disorders. Follow-up had shown that children of higher intelligence, though severely handicapped by impairment of motor skills, might improve remarkably with increasing maturation and eventually benefit from normal education. The more severely affected children of average or below average intelligence require specialised training from teachers fully versed with their problems. It was apparent that a discrepancy between the Verbal and Performance IQ scores of the WISC was an important confirmatory test in recognising such cases, supplemented by a battery of other psychological tests designed to assess executive and cognitive skills. It seemed necessary that the existence of a syndrome of specific clumsiness should be made more widely known so that it could be recognised earlier and more appropriately managed.

This Newcastle study engendered further interest in the delineation of Developmental Clumsiness by providing the basis of a survey of motor abilities in a cross section of Western Australian schoolchildren. Chapters 4 and 5 describe the survey in detail and also the development of simple standardised tests of motor ability which are offered for general use in the assessment of children.

SUMMARY AND CONCLUSIONS

A group of 21 children presenting with severe clumsiness and poor school performance have been described in detail. All of the children manifested cognitive and performance defects which could be classified as various forms of apraxia and agnosia. Seven of the subjects showed minor collateral evidence of brain dysfunction including minimal signs of pyramidal or cerebellar dysfunction which were not sufficiently severe to cause their clumsiness. Fourteen of the children had apraxic and agnosic disorders in isolation and some of these exhibited abnormal movements which resembled those of chorea; these have been discussed in detail.

The aetiology of the syndrome has been discussed; the possibilities include inadequate establishment of cerebral dominance, delayed maturation, and structural lesions in one or the other parietal lobe. It is possible that the 14 children with 'pure' executive or cognitive defects are a heterogenous group with respect to aetiology; however, electroencephalographic evidence and a high incidence of perinatal abnormality suggests that underlying organic structural disturbance is usually present. Nevertheless, the possibility that in some cases the condition is due to defective establishment of brain dominance in a physiological rather than an anatomical sense cannot be denied; there was evidence of 'crossed laterality' in at least seven cases.

While some of the more intelligent children improved markedly with maturation, they often demonstrated behaviour disorders early in school life due to the failure of teachers to recognise the nature of their difficulties. The more severely affected children of average or below average intelligence required patient and individual tuition from teachers specially trained to deal with these cases. The existence of the syndrome should be more widely known so that it can be recognised earlier and more effective methods of management sought. Thus there is a need for the development of convenient, standardised tests of motor ability which would facilitate the recognition of 'clumsy children'.

CHAPTER FOUR

A Survey of Developmental Clumsiness in Schoolchildren

Before embarking on a full survey of motor performance in schoolchildren in Perth, Western Australia, it was considered necessary to conduct a pilot survey for two principal reasons. Firstly, a battery of tests, standardised for age, was needed for the rapid selection of children who fell into the lowest range of motor performance, and secondly, a 'trial run' seemed highly desirable before planning the complicated operation of efficiently obtaining the co-operation of teachers and schoolchildren alike. It was realised that a more accurate standardisation of tests would be forthcoming after the completion of the total survey and in fact this was one of the fundamental aims of the entire study. The salient findings of this pilot survey have been reported elsewhere (Gubbay and Stenhouse, 1973). There were similarities between the approach to this study and that reported by Rutter, Tizard and Whitmore (1970) in a comprehensive series of surveys in education, health and behaviour of 9- to 12-year-old children in the defined geographical area of the Isle of Wight, England.

The WL Primary State School was selected for the pilot survey because it offered sufficient pupils to meet the requirements of a statistically valid study and was in close proximity to Princess Margaret Hospital for Children where electroencephalographic examinations were to be carried out. Excellent facilities for the purpose of the study were provided at the school. There was also a wide academic spectrum of children, particularly as there were two special classes (senior and junior) for children with specific educational problems.

At first, all the children attending the school were examined, but eventually the survey was narrowed to 279 of the 327 children on the school roll (see Table 4.1). They ranged in age from 6 years 0 months to 12 years 11 months. Apart from absentees, the children excluded from the survey were younger or older than these age limits or were recent immigrants from Europe and were unable to communicate adequately in English.

94

Each class teacher was supplied with a questionnaire (see below) which requested basic information regarding each child including age, sex and the total time that the child had been under the particular schoolteacher's observation. They were asked to comment on the child's handwriting, sporting ability, and tendency to clumsiness and fidgetiness. Additional information regarding the child's general conduct and popularity with schoolmates was sought in the questionnaire. The questionnaires were answered conscientiously and the results were used as a basis for comparison with both assessments by parents and objective assessments elicited through specific tests of motor ability.

QUESTIONNAIRE FOR CLASS TEACHER

Name of School (Initials) .... Date ....
Name of Schoolteacher: Mr: Mrs: Miss: ....
Grade of Class: ....
Name of Child (Block letters): ....
                              Surname   First Name
Address: .... (Post Code)
Date of birth: Day: .... Month: .... Year: 19 ....
Age: .... years   .... months
Sex: Male .... Female ....
How many months ago did this child first come under your observation?

Put tick in appropriate space below:
1. Is the formation and neatness of this child's handwriting much below average?
              No .... Possible .... Yes ....
2. Is the child's sporting ability and bodily agility much below average?
              No .... Possible .... Yes ....
3. Is the child unduly clumsy?
              No .... Possible .... Yes ....
4. Does the child fidget excessively in class?
              No .... Possible .... Yes ....
5. Is the child's conduct much below average?
              No .... Possible .... Yes ....
6. Is the child unpopular with schoolmates?
              No .... Possible .... Yes ....

Each child was examined singly with a battery of 17 tests of motor performance (see below) which were to be used as the basis of the final tests employed for the identification of clumsy children. It was considered expedient at this stage to include tests which were not specifically of motor performance, but which would provide valuable data for correlative purposes. These extra tests incorporated the assessment of manual and pedal dominance as well as stereognosis, finger sense, right–left orientation, and the ability to copy certain finger postures (test items 14 to 17 inclusive). In order to obtain further information which could be correlated with tests of agility and dexterity, additional group examinations were devised where the children were examined classroom by classroom with tests of handwriting and drawing.

The results of the valid items of tests of motor performance in the schoolchildren were tabulated and the children who scored roughly within the lowest 10 per cent of their age group were identified. These children were considered to have 'failed' the tests and the children with the largest numbers of failures were selected out from each age group and identified as 'clumsy children', when they were submitted to further analysis. This method of selection was approximate, but its validity was verified later by the more objective methods of statistical analysis.

The 'clumsy children' were matched for age and sex with control children whose individual surnames alphabetically followed those of the 'clumsy children' in the same classroom. Thus 19 'clumsy children' and 19 controls were obtained from the school. Parental approval was sought before submitting the children firstly to full neurological and general examinations and secondly to electroencephalographic examination. Approval was obtained for the examination in 35 out of the 38 children so selected.

INDIVIDUAL SCREENING EXAMINATION

The tests of motor ability were in three broad categories comprising: (1) facial and lingual praxis; (2) trunk and leg praxis; and (3) manual praxis. The first group included the child's ability to close the eyes and protrude the tongue simultaneously; and to wink one eye and whistle independently. A child was considered to have failed with the 'winking' test if he were unable to see out of the contralateral eye at the time of winking and was considered to have failed with the 'whistle' test if a musical note could not be emitted even momentarily (Items 1 and 2).

In the second group of tests, the child was expected to hop on his preferred (dominant) leg 10 times in a straight line indicated on the ground; and to walk heel to toe in 'tandem' fashion along the line (Figure 4.1). If necessary, each child was allowed three attempts to carry out these tests (Items 3 and 4) which had to be performed without adjustments of the feet or stepping off the line. Item 5 consisted of making five successive skips allowing for three attempts, and if necessary after a demonstration by the examiner. Item 6 tested the child's ability to roll a tennis ball under the dominant foot in a spiral fashion around six matchboxes (Figure 4.2) whilst attempting to oppose the sole of the foot continually to the top of the ball without kicking it. A child who repeatedly lost control of the ball was given a maximum of three attempts at the test before being considered to have failed it. This latter test was timed with a stopwatch as were most of the following tests of manual dexterity. The click of the stopwatch indicated the start of each timed test.

The third group of tests, those relating to manual praxis which were also timed in seconds, included tying one shoelace of the examiner with a double bow (Item 9), threading 10 beads (Item 10), piercing 20 pinholes along two rows of adjacent 1/10 inch (0.25 cm) squares of graph paper (Item 11) and placing six coloured plastic objects of variable shape into appropriate slots in

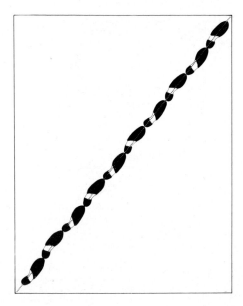

Figure 4.1. Individual Screening Examination Item 4. Walking 10 steps heel to toe in a straight line. Reproduced with the kind permission of the editor of *Neurology* (India).

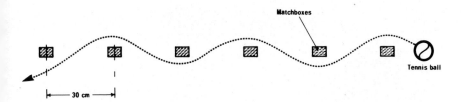

Figure 4.2. Individual Screening Examination Item 6. Rolling a tennis ball in a spiral around 6 matchboxes. Reproduced with the kind permission of the editors of *Neurology* (India), and *Proceedings of the Australian Association of Neurologists*.

the fashion of a 'form board' (posting box—Item 13). The wooden beads were 3.0 cm in diameter and contained a central hole whose bore was 0.8 cm (Figure 4.3). The child was expected to thread each bead individually with the preferred hand as fast as possible on to a stiffened string 0.3 cm in diameter. 'Kiddicraft' Toy Beads were used for the bead-threading test (Figure 4.4). A hatpin measuring 10 cm in length was used as the stylus for piercing the holes in graph paper (Figure 4.5). The 'Kiddicraft' posting box toy was used for the test requiring visuomotor co-ordination (Figure 4.6a, b).

A further test of manual dexterity and timing consisted of catching a tennis ball after throwing it up into the air and clapping the hands (Item 8). The more dexterous children were able to clap their hands more times before catching the

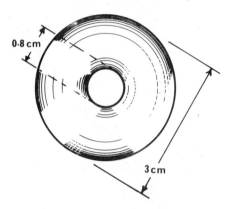

Figure 4.3. Individual Screening Examination Item 10. Diagram showing dimensions of wooden bead (see Figure 4.4). Reproduced with the kind permission of the editors of *Neurology* (India), and *Proceedings of the Australian Association of Neurologists*.

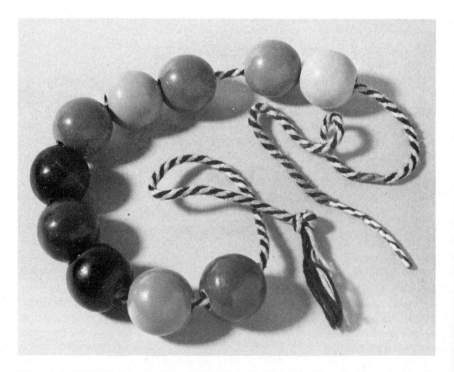

Figure 4.4. Individual Screening Examination Item 10. Threading 10 beads. Reproduced with the kind permission of the editors of *Neurology* (India), and *Proceedings of the Australian Association of Neurologists*.

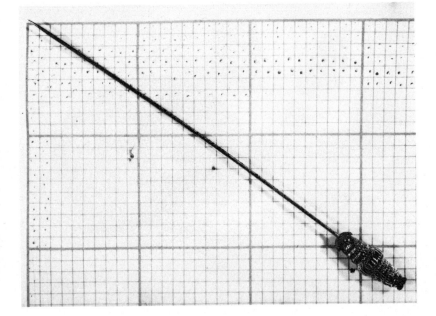

Figure 4.5. Individual Screening Examination Item 11. Piercing 20 pinholes along two adjacent rows in graph paper. Reproduced with the kind permission of the editors of *Neurology* (India), and *Proceedings of the Australian Association of Neurologists*.

ball and the most dexterous of all were able to catch the ball with only one (the dominant) hand. The child was not asked to clap the hands more than four times before catching the ball and each child was allowed three attempts before failing at any particular point.

In the test of stereognosis (Item 14), the child was given a cloth bag measuring 33 cm in depth by 27 cm in width which contained eight articles including comb, key, matchbox, toothbrush, coat button, safety pin, bottle top and pencil (Figure 4.7). The child was asked to turn his head away and close the eyes. He was to extricate each object singly, as quickly as possible and verbally identify them in turn. If the child did not nominate every object correctly, he was considered to have failed the test; otherwise the total time taken for the test was recorded.

Finger praxis (Item 15) was tested by asking each child to copy three separate finger postures with the dominant hand as demonstrated by the examiner. These included: (a) protruding the thumb between the index and middle fingers with the palm closed; (b) crossing of the middle finger over the index finger; and (c) abducting the middle finger from the ring finger with all the other digits adducted (Figure 4.8a, b, c).

Although not strictly tests of motor performance, there were also simple screening tests of appreciation of body image and of extrapersonal space. The

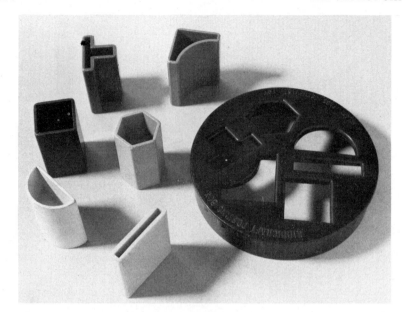

(a)

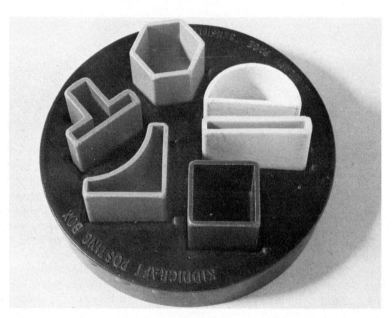

(b)

Figure 4.6. a. Individual Screening Examination Item 13. The posting box before insertion of objects. b. The posting box after insertion of objects. Reproduced with the kind permission of the editors of *Neurology* (India), and *Proceedings of the Australian Association of Neurologists*.

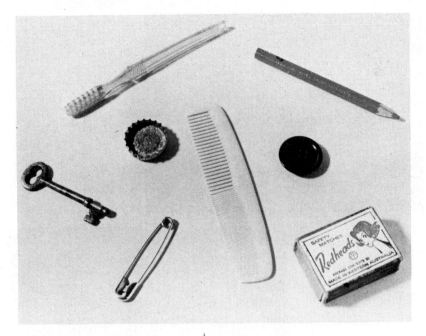

Figure 4.7. Individual Screening Examination Item 14. Articles used for stereognosis. Reproduced with the kind permission of the editor of *Neurology* (India).

first of these was a test of finger sense employing the 'in-between' test of Kinsbourne and Warrington (1962) and using the subject's dominant hand (Item 16). Two of the subject's digits were touched by the examiner, and with eyes closed the subject was required to state the number of fingers 'in-between' the two that were touched. A sequence of five subtests was employed (Figure 4.9):

	Finger touched	*Number 'in-between'*
A	Thumb and ring	2
B	Middle and little	1
C	Thumb and little	3
D	Thumb and middle	1
E	Index and middle	0

A score was given corresponding to the number of correct answers by the child. The second of these series of tests was for right–left orientation (Item 17) and included three subtests as follows:

1. Raise your left hand!
2. Touch your right hand on your left ear!
3. Touch my left elbow with your right hand!

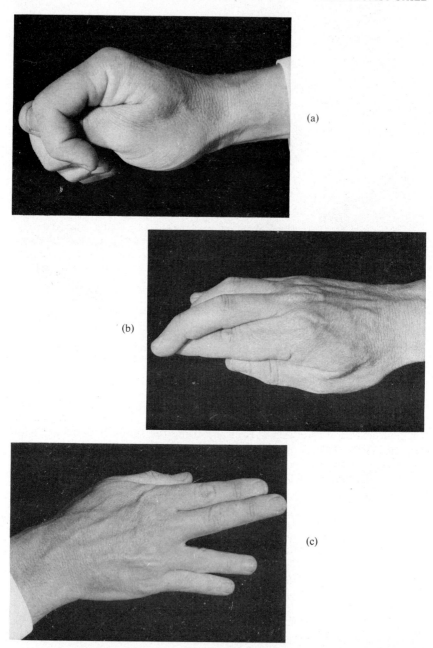

(a)

(b)

(c)

Figure 4.8. a. Individual Screening Examination Item 15. Tests of finger praxis—protruding thumb between index and middle fingers ('thumb between' test). b. Tests of finger praxis—crossing middle finger over index finger ('cross fingers' test). c. Tests of finger praxis—abducting middle finger from ring finger with other digits adducted ('benediction' test).

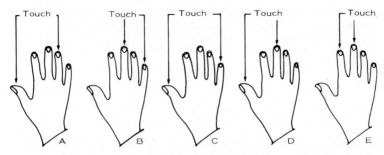

Figure 4.9. Individual Screening Examination Item 16. 'In-between' test. The subject was asked to state the number of digits 'in-between' the two that were touched.

The child was tested until the point of failure, i.e. if he raised his right hand for the first test, the second and third tests were not given. One point was given for subtest 1, and two points each for subtests 2 and 3, allowing a possible total of five points.

The proforma used for the individual screening examination is shown below:

INDIVIDUAL SCREENING EXAMINATION

$\sqrt{}$ = success   X = failure

Name .... Date.............

Click of stopwatch indicates start in timed tests.

1. Close your eyes and poke out your tongue!
2. Wink one eye and whistle!
3. Hop on dominant leg 10 times without error (3 attempts)!
4. Walk heel to toe along line without adjustment (3 attempts)!
5. Make 5 successive skips (3 attempts after demonstration)!
6. Roll ball with dominant foot in spiral around 6 matchboxes!
   (3 attempts—no touching).   .... secs
7. Foot dominance   R   L   RL
8. Throw ball up, clap hands up to 4 times then catch both hands or dominant hand
   (3 attempts)!
   Can't catch   0   1   2   3   4   4D
9. Tie both shoelaces with double bow!   .... secs
10. Thread 10 beads!   .... secs
11. Pierce 20 holes in graph paper!   .... secs
12. Hand Dominance   R   L   RL
13. Posting Box   .... secs
14. Stereognosis (8 articles hidden in bag—comb, key, matchbox, toothbrush, coat button, safety pin, bottle top, pencil.
    .... correct   .... secs

15. Copy finger postures (1) 'thumb between' (2) 'cross fingers' (3) 'benediction'.
16. Finger sense (dominant hand)—'in between' 2, 1, 3, 1, 0 (out of 5).
17. Raise your left hand!
     Touch your right hand on your left ear!
     Touch my left elbow with your right hand!

GROUP SCREENING EXAMINATION

This examination was administered to each classroom group collectively. Each child was issued with a specially ruled sheet of quarto paper (Figure 4.10) and a grade 2B (soft) lead pencil. Firstly, they were asked to write (not print) their names and addresses in appropriate areas. Secondly, they were directed to write to dictation 'The quick brown fox jumps over the lazy dog'. Each subject was required to write the following numbers in numerals; 12; 345; 6079. Sufficient time was given to complete these tests and no erasing was permitted. It was anticipated in this manner that dyslexic subjects might be detected. The lower half of the quarto sheet issued to each child was ruled into six equal areas. In the top left-hand area the children were asked to draw a circle. After sufficient time was allowed for all to finish, they were asked to insert the numbers of a clock-face from 1 to 12. Again sufficient time was allowed before the children were instructed to mark the time at 10 minutes to 2 o'clock. Finally, they were given 60 seconds to copy five geometric figures as far as possible in the five remaining rectangles on their test paper.

FOLLOW-UP NEUROLOGICAL AND EEG EXAMINATION

After submitting all the children to the individual screening and group screening examinations, the clumsiest 10 per cent of the entire school were selected according to criteria stated earlier in this chapter. The parents of the 19 children and 19 controls were interviewed in order to obtain permission for clinical examination and EEG after explaining the purpose of the study. The parents completed a questionnaire supplying the relevant medical, developmental and social background of each child. The Questionnaire for Parents is produced later in the chapter in the description of the definitive survey.

After approval, 35 of the 38 children (17 clumsy and 18 control children) were subjected to neurological and general examination. Each child was also asked to assess his or her own health, including the tendency to headache, faints or fits. Their own individual subjective assessment of sporting ability was also obtained and the reading age was evaluated according to Reading Test R 1 of Schonell and Schonell (1950). The skull circumference of each child was measured and the skull contour noted. All cranial nerve functions were examined and, in the limbs, tone, power, abnormal movements, co-ordination, deep reflexes, superficial reflexes and sensation were assessed. Each child was also subjected to a general examination including the respiratory and cardiovascular systems and abdominal palpation, together with a blood

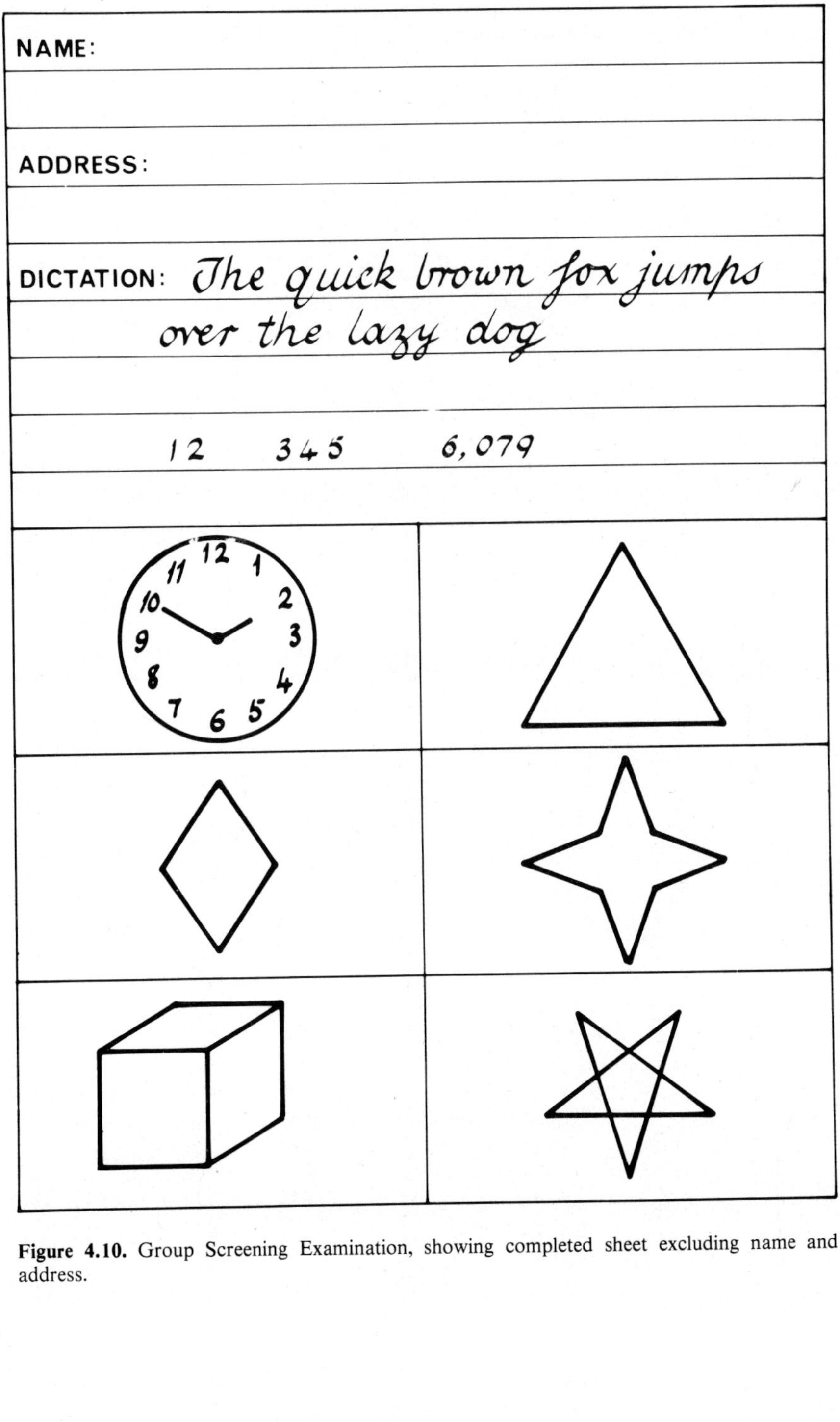
NAME:

ADDRESS:

DICTATION: The quick brown fox jumps over the lazy dog

12 345 6,079

Figure 4.10. Group Screening Examination, showing completed sheet excluding name and address.

pressure recording, and obvious congenital abnormalities were noted. Speech function was appraised in greater detail particularly for evidence of stammer or articulatory disturbances. Finally, the child's co-operation and tendency to hyperactivity were noted.

Electroencephalographic examinations were carried out on all the 17 clumsy and 18 control children evaluated neurologically. The recordist was unaware of the category to which each child belonged and was asked to comment only on the amount of eye movement and muscle potential artifact in the recordings.

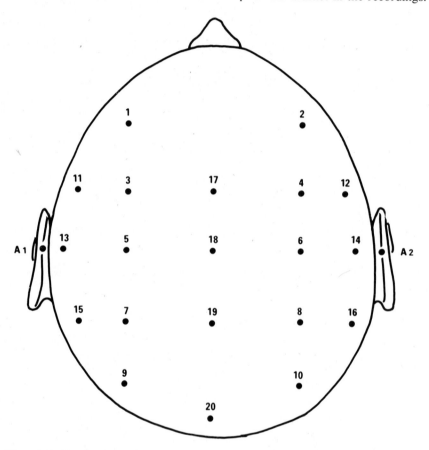

Figure 4.11. The six unipolar runs. A1 and A2 represent left and right 'indifferent' ear electrodes

Channel	Run 1	Run 2	Run 3	Run 4	Run 5	Run 6
1	1−A1	1−A2	7−A1	7−A2	9−A1	9−A2
2	2−A2	2−A1	8−A2	8−A1	10−A2	10−A1
3	5−A1	5−A2	11−A1	11−A2	13−A1	13−A2
4	6−A2	6−A1	12−A2	12−A1	14−A2	14−A1
5	9−A1	9−A2	13−A1	13−A2	15−A1	15−A2
6	10−A2	10−A1	14−A2	14−A1	16−A2	16−A1
7	13−A1	13−A2	15−A1	15−A2	18−A1	18−A2
8	14−A2	14−A1	16−A2	16−A1	A1−A2	A1−A2

She was asked to note the child's medication if any, examine a specimen of urine from each for sugar and albumin and record the height and weight.

Recordings were obtained from the children in the resting, awake state for 20 minutes; during hyperventilation for 3 minutes; and during photic stimulation with 1, double, 5, 10, 15 and 20 flashes per second. It was not possible to obtain many sleep studies because of the heavy routine clinical load on the department. The scalp electrodes were placed according to a modified

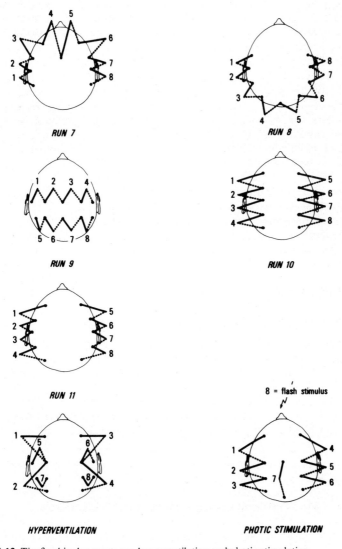

Figure 4.12. The five bipolar montages, hyperventilation and photic stimulation.

international '10–20 system' and recordings were made with a 'Grass' 8-channel electroencephalograph. Six unipolar and seven bipolar montages including separate hyperventilation and photic stimulation runs were used for each child. The ear was employed as the 'indifferent' electrode in the unipolar tracings. The 2nd, 4th and 6th runs were duplicates of the 1st, 3rd and 5th runs respectively except for alteration of the indifferent ear electrode to the opposite side. Thus in runs 1, 3 and 5 electrical potentials were recorded between left-sided scalp electrodes and the left earlobe in 4 channels, and between right-sided scalp electrodes and the right earlobe in the other 4. The even runs 2, 4 and 6 employed the contralateral ears for the indifferent electrodes (Figure 4.11). The five bipolar montages (runs 7 to 11), hyperventilation montage (run 12) and photic stimulation montage (run 13) are represented diagrammatically in Figure 4.12.

Each of the electroencephalograms was examined personally when only the age of the child was available and without knowledge of the identity or category of the subject in order to reduce observer bias. At this stage the results were tabulated according to the proforma shown later in this chapter. The factors for assessment included organisation, dominant anterior and posterior rhythms, amplitudes of alpha activity on either side and the tendency for alpha blockade with eye opening. The full range of frequencies was determined with special reference to paroxysmal theta and paroxysmal delta activity. Spike and paroxysmal spike-wave activity was noted. Finally, the response to hyperventilation and photic stimulation including the production of sharp, spike or paroxysmal activity was estimated.

The proformas used for the Neurological and General Examination and the Electroencephalogram are shown later in the chapter in the description of the Total (Definitive) Survey.

RESULTS OF THE PILOT SURVEY

These results are considered in four sections as follows:

Section A: Selection of clumsy children and their controls
Section B: Comparison of the observations on the 19 clumsy children and 19 controls in the teachers' questionnaires and screening examinations.
Section C: Comparison of the follow-up observations on 17 clumsy children and 18 controls (three subjects of the 38 defaulted to follow-up).
Section D: Mechanism of standardisation of screening tests for the total survey.

RESULTS

Section A: The Selection of Clumsy Children and Their Controls

All children at the school between the ages of 6 years 0 months and 12 years 11 months were included in this study (Table 4.1). Originally 12 children

Table 4.1. Total number of children in each age group

Age				Male	Female	Total
6 years 0 months to		6 years 11 months		17	19	36
7	0	to 7	11	15	20	35
8	0	to 8	11	16	14	30
9	0	to 9	11	28	17	45
10	0	to 10	11	18	28	46
11	0	to 11	11	23	24	47
12	0	to 12	11	20	20	40
6	0	to 12	11	137	142	279

altogether in the 13-year-old group were examined, but they were excluded later from the study except for a male aged 13 years 2 months who was initially selected as a control because of the closest proximity of his age to that of a clumsy child in his own classroom. The 13-year-olds were an atypical group which represented children who were over-age for primary school. Two hundred and forty-five of the children had been under the observation of their individual schoolteachers completing the questionnaire for up to 9 months (representing one academic year) and 35 children for more than 9 months. Thus 279 children were studied between the ages of 6 years 0 months and 12 years 11 months. The children in the six- and seven-year-old groups were excluded later from analysis in the pilot survey because it became obvious that the screening tests employed were not sufficiently critical in this age group. Therefore the clumsy children and their controls were selected from the 208 children in the 8- to 12-year-old age groups inclusive. The clumsy children were all within one year in age of their individual controls.

Section B: Comparison of the Observations on the 19 Clumsy Children and 19 Controls in the Teachers' Questionnaires and Screening Examinations

The sex, age and schoolclass distribution are given in Table 4.2.

Teachers' questionnaire

The teacher of each class in the survey was asked six questions relating to each child and was required to answer 'yes', 'no' or 'possible' to each question. These results are given in Table 4.3.

All the results show a definite trend towards a more inferior performance in the clumsy group than in the control group according to the schoolteachers' observations. The difference reaches statistical significance in the category where very poor ability at sport and undue clumsiness ('yes' or 'possible') is compared ($P < 0.05$). If the total number of 'yes' answers is compared in the two groups, the differences are statistically significant ($P < 0.05$), but the difference is highly significant ($P < 0.001$) when the 43 'yes' or 'possible' answers in the clumsy group are compared with the 17 in the controls.

Table 4.2. Sex, age and schoolclass distribution

	Clumsy	Controls
Male	8	7
Female	11	12
Age range	8 years 2 months to 12 years 11 months	8 years 6 months to 13 years 2 months
Years old:		
8	4	3
9	4	5
10	3	3
11	3	4
12	5	3
13	0	1
Average age:	10 years 5 months	10 years 7 months
Grade:		
2	2	0
3	4	3
4	4	7
5	1	0
6	3	5
7	0	3
Junior special	2	0
Senior special	3	1

The special classes were for children with learning problems.

Table 4.3. Answers in teachers' questionnaires

	Clumsy			Controls		
	No	Possible	Yes	No	Possible	Yes
Q1 Handwriting	12	2	5	15	1	3
Q2 Sport	9	4	6	16	2	1
Q3 Clumsy	11	6	2	16	2	1
Q4 Fidgety	13	4	2	17	0	2
Q5 Conduct	16	1	2	16	3	0
Q6 Unpopular	15	3	1	17	2	0
Handwriting	3 No's	2 No's	1 No	0 No's	3 No's	2 No's	1 No	0 No's
Sport and Clumsy	7	3	5	4	15	1	0	3

	Clumsy	Controls
Sport and Clumsy	Yes for either or both	5	1
Sport and Clumsy	Yes or possible for either or both	11	3 $P < 0.05$
Total Yes Answers Q1–Q6		19	7 $P < 0.05$
Total Yes or Possible Q1–Q6		43	17 $P < 0.001$

Individual and group screening examinations

Not all the tests in the individual screening examination questionnaire were designed to select clumsy children, as some were to be used for correlative purposes. Statistically significant differences were found in the performances of 19 clumsy children as compared with 19 controls in the following test items:

1. Ability to whistle ($P < 0.01$)
2. Roll ball in spiral around 6 matchboxes ($P < 0.01$)
3. Throw ball up, clap hands and catch ($P < 0.01$)
4. Thread 10 beads ($P < 0.001$)
5. Pierce 20 holes in paper ($P < 0.01$)
6. Posting box ($P < 0.001$)
7. Finger sense—less than four correct ($P < 0.05$)
8. Writing to dictation with no mistakes ($P < 0.01$)
9. Ability to insert clock hands at designated time ($P < 0.01$).

In all the other test items there was an obvious trend towards superior performance in the control children, but one which did not reach statistical significance.

In actual fact the clumsy children had been selected on the basis of their inferior performance in tests which showed a good degree of differentiation between the clumsiest children and all the others in the pilot trial. The above analysis which shows a statistical significance between the performance in the clumsy children as compared with their controls should be regarded therefore as axiomatic. However, the analysis does serve to show the relative reliability of each of the test items.

Section C: Comparison of the Follow-up Observations on 17 Clumsy Children and 18 Controls

Two of the 19 clumsy children and one of the 19 controls defaulted to the follow-up examinations consisting of:

1. Parents' questionnaire
2. Neurological examination
3. Group intelligence tests
4. Electroencephalogram.

It is unnecessary to consider the comparison between the above follow-up examinations between the clumsy children and their controls in detail at this stage as they are considered later in the chapter when incorporated into the rest of the data from the definitive total survey. A basic reason for carrying out this pilot survey was to confirm that the children identified as 'clumsy' by the devised screening tests were also clumsy in the estimation of their parents. It was also of major interest, before carrying out the definitive survey, to know whether the clumsy group exhibited a higher incidence of abnormalities in the neurological examination and EEG and that they were of normal intelligence.

There was a good response from the parents regarding approval of detailed

physical and EEG examination (35 out of 38 children). There were some
missing data in the parents' questionnaires which might have been predicted as
many parents were unwilling to commit themselves to a definite answer (e.g. 'at
which age did your child first learn to speak in sentences') even if they could
clearly remember that their child's performance was normal. The questions
were rephrased therefore in the rest of the Total Survey where specifically
affirmative or negative answers were sought on the proformas (see Parents'
Questionnaire).

Validation of screening tests for clumsiness

Nine of the 17 clumsy children and only one of the 18 controls were
considered to be:

1. 'unduly clumsy' by their schoolteachers
2. and/or 'much below average in sporting ability and bodily agility' by their
   schoolteachers
3. and/or 'much below average in ability at sporting activity' by their parents
4. and/or 'very clumsy in his or her movements' by their parents
5. and/or 'much below average in sporting ability' by themselves.

Thus:

Clumsy children with significant reported problems = 9
Control children with significant reported problems = 1

These results were very significant ($P < 0.01$) and confirmed the validity of
the selection of the clumsy children by the screening test devised. As it
transpired, the only control child with reported problems was in the borderline
clumsy range. There was a higher degree of correlation between the screening
test results and the schoolteachers' assessments than between the screening
tests and the parents' or children's assessments.

Electroencephalograms

The results of the individual EEG observations again are not considered in
detail at this stage as they are embodied in the total data in the definitive
survey. Table 4.4 summarises the general conclusions regarding the EEG
appearances. There were 10 abnormal records out of 17 tracings in the clumsy
children and 3 out of the 18 in the controls ($P < 0.05$).

Table 4.4. EEG abnormalities

Category of abnormality	Clumsy (total 17)	Control (total 18)
Normal	7	15
Borderline abnormal	1	1
Mildly abnormal	7	1
Moderately abnormal	2	1
Grossly abnormal	0	0
Totally abnormal	10	3

Reproduced with the kind permission of the editor of *Neurology* (India).

Section D: The Mechanism of the Standardisation of the Screening Tests for the Total Survey

The validity of the screening tests used for the identification of clumsy children had been ratified by the joint observations of the parents, teachers and children involved. It was now justifiable to determine a set of standard values for the same screening tests to be used in the total survey. Only the 8- to 12-year-old standards were determined as the tests proved unsuitable for application to six- and seven-year-olds. The detailed methods regarding the standards used for test failures are fully described by Gubbay (1972) and are only briefly discussed here. The general conclusions regarding the individual original screening tests are given below.

Close eyes and protrude tongue simultaneously. As each child passed this combined test it was therefore deleted from the total survey because it had no discriminatory value.

Wink preferred eye. The results were very unreliable and the test was therefore deleted from the total survey.

Whistle through pouted lips. The performance with this test improved with increasing age. The test was retained as it seemed a fairly reliable overall index of faciolingual motor maturity. It was appreciated that the test might show a sex difference because girls tend to be discouraged from whistling in their normal environment.

Hop on dominant leg 10 times. There was such a high degree of success with this test that it had no discriminative value in the age groups and was therefore deleted from the total survey screening examinations, but retained as part of the supplementary neurological examination as hopping is so frequently tested in routine neurological examinations in children.

Walk heel to toe 10 steps. Only one 12-year-old child failed this test which was deleted from further screening examinations but retained for the supplementary neurological examination.

Skip five times. Ten out of 204 children could not skip (5 per cent) and the distribution and percentage of failures suggested that this test would be useful to retain for the total survey.

Clap hands before catching ball. The generally improving performance with increasing age rendered this standardised test ideal for the selection of clumsy children in the total survey.

Tie shoelaces, Thread 10 beads, Pierce 20 holes in graph paper, Posting box. These four timed tests were retained because there was a good differentiation in all age groups between clumsy and control children. All children who took longer than 23 seconds to tie shoelaces were in fact not able to do so within 60 seconds and were classed as test failures.

Stereognosis. As a timed test, stereognosis was found to be quite unreliable because its unweildiness allowed for excessive variables within the test situation. Hence the test was deleted from the total survey screening examination, but retained for the supplementary neurological examination.

Copy finger postures. The 'thumb between' and 'cross fingers' tests were too simple and the 'benediction' test too difficult in all age groups to be of discriminative value and therefore all were deleted from the total survey screening examination, but retained in the supplementary neurological examination.

Finger sense and right–left orientation. The tests were not intended as true screening tests, but they were retained for later correlative information in the supplementary neurological examination.

On the basis of the foregoing data it was concluded that the eight screening tests worth retaining for the total survey were:

1. Whistle through pouted lips
2. Make five successive skips (3 attempts after demonstration)
3. Roll ball with dominant foot in spiral around 6 matchboxes at 30-cm intervals (3 attempts—no touching)
4. Throw ball up, clap hands up to 4 times and catch both hands or dominant hand (3 attempts)
5. Tie single shoelace with double bow
6. Thread 10 beads
7. Pierce 20 holes in graph paper
8. Posting box.

The standardised failure levels (i.e. tenth percentile levels) of each age group are given in Table 4.5. For convenience, the mean tenth percentile values were then adopted as the overall standard for the entire age range of 8 to 12 years to be used in the total survey.

It was noted that the overall standard tenth percentile values were almost identical to the tenth percentiles determined for the 10-year-olds.

In applying the new criteria of failure in the eight screening tests (Table 4.6) it was obviously necessary to have an inverse relationship between the number of test failures and the age of the child in the selection of clumsy children in the total survey (Table 4.7).

With the retrospective application of these new criteria it was found that:

1. Only three further clumsy children would have been identified and these three were in a borderline category in any case.
2. Thirteen of the 19 clumsy children originally selected in the pilot survey would now qualify as clumsy for the total survey. The rest of the clumsy children were 'borderline clumsy' or those who had been selected on the unreliable stereognosis test which was now discarded.
3. There were 16 clumsy children out of 208 8- to 12-year-olds at the school (Table 4.8).

Table 4.5. Standardised failure levels (per cent) for total survey

	Age (years)										Overall standard failure level
	8		9		10		11		12		
Whistle	Failure	52	Failure	27	Failure	26	Failure	17	Failure	15	Failure
Skip	Failure	3	Failure	2	Failure	5	Failure	9	Failure	5	Failure
Roll ball	>22 sec	16	>18 sec	11	>18 sec	22	>18 sec	9	>18 sec	8	>18 sec
Clap-catch	<2 claps	10	<3 claps	30	<3 claps	9	<3 claps	11	<3 claps	10	<3 claps
Shoelaces	>23 sec	19	>15 sec	11	>13 sec	9	>13 sec	13	>13 sec	10	>15 sec
Beads	>45 sec	10	>42 sec	11	>38 sec	11	>36 sec	11	>36 sec	13	>38 sec
Holes	>38 sec	10	>25 sec	11	>24 sec	13	>18 sec	9	>18 sec	28	>24 sec
Post box	>25 sec	10	>18 sec	11	>18 sec	9	>18 sec	11	>18 sec	18	>18 sec

Table 4.6. New criteria of failure in 8 screening tests

Test		Failure
1. Whistle	=	Failure
2. Skip 5 times	=	Failure
3. Roll ball	=	>18 sec
4. Clap-catch ball	=	< 3 claps
5. Tie shoelace	=	>15 sec
6. Thread 10 beads	=	>38 sec
7. Pierce 20 holes	=	>24 sec
8. Posting box	=	>18 sec

Reproduced with the kind permission of the editors of *Neurology* (India) and *Proceedings of the Australian Association of Neurologists*.

Table 4.7. New criteria of selection of clumsy child

Age	No. of failures
8	6
9	5
10	4
11	3
12	2

Reproduced with the kind permission of the editor of *Neurology* (India).

Table 4.8. Number of failures in each age group (new criteria)

Age	0	1	2	3	4	5	6	7	8	Total in each age group
8	2	5	5	6	5	5	2	0	0	30
9	15	15	8	2	3	2	0	0	0	45
10	19	17	6	0	3	0	0	1	0	46
11	22	19	4	2	0	0	0	0	0	47
12	25	9	2	0	2	0	1	0	1	40
										208

The 16 clumsy children's results appear on the right side of the oblique line.

THE TOTAL (DEFINITIVE) SURVEY

The experience and facts gained from the pilot survey permitted greater efficiency in the subsequent collection of data. The standardised tests for the selection of clumsy children determined a far more confident approach to the task of screening the 8- to 12-year-old population of four further schools. Experience had also crystallised the method of approach to school authorities, parents and children. The principal findings have been recorded previously by Gubbay (1972, 1973, 1975).

Altogether, 922 children were screened in the five schools involved in the total survey. Nine hundred and nineteen of these children were aged 8 to 12 years inclusive at the date of screening, i.e. they had reached their eighth birthday, but not their 13th birthday on the date of testing. All pupils in remedial classes were included and the only exclusions were absentees and children who had obvious physical encumbrances (e.g. healing limb fractures) which would invalidate their test performance. Fortunately all the schools' principals appreciated the innocuous nature of the screening tests and used their discretion to facilitate unimpeded access to the children without reference to parental approval. There was no modification of the original selection of schools as all the school principals who were approached gave their approval.

The total of the five school populations was necessary to ensure a statistically valid representation of children of each sex and age group from differing sociocultural levels. The five schools examined were:

1. WLSS (government mixed primary school—pilot survey)
2. LSS (government mixed primary school)
3. PMS (government mixed secondary school)
4. CCGS (private boys' primary and secondary school)
5. SHS (private girls' primary and secondary school).

The first three schools, namely WLSS, LSS and PMS, were all within a mile of each other and of Princess Margaret Hospital for Children where the electroencephalograms were carried out. These institutions drew their pupils from the local suburban populations consisting largely of labourers, white collar workers and tradesmen with only occasional professional groups. Many of their families were recent immigrants from the United Kingdom and Italy. The children from the two private schools were largely from socially privileged homes with a high proportion of professional and successful business backgrounds.

It was intended, firstly, to collect normative data which would permit the final standardisation of the screening tests and secondly, to compare the information relating to the clumsy children and their controls. Thus, this study had set out to achieve an objective method of rapid recognition of clumsy children as well as to provide further information about their characteristics.

Method

The method used in the pilot survey on WLSS was modified and then applied to the remaining four schools in identical fashion. The children of one school were all given the screening examination before proceeding to the next school. Correlative data regarding each child were also obtained from his or her schoolteacher. The clumsy children were selected after completing the screening examination on all the schools. An equal number of control children were selected in the same fashion as in the pilot survey. Finally, all the clumsy and control children were subjected to detailed physical, electro-encephalographic and IQ examinations.

The work proformas used in the pilot survey were only slightly modified for the total survey. Each of the school principals preferred to use his or her own discretion regarding the wording of the letters to parents requesting approval for physical examination and EEG, but the substance of each letter was the same.

The questionnaire for teachers

The teachers' questionnaire differed from that used in the pilot survey in only one modification consisting of the additional question 'Is this child's overall academic performance much below average for his/her age?' The question was added to determine whether academic failure might be correlated with clumsiness. The complete format of the questionnaire is not reproduced here, but the seven principal questions are listed below. An answer was required in one of the three categories, namely 'yes', 'no' or 'possible':

1. Is the formation and neatness of this child's handwriting much below average?
2. Is the child's sporting ability and bodily agility much below average?
3. Is the child unduly clumsy?
4. Does the child fidget excessively in class?
5. Is the child's conduct much below average?
6. Is the child unpopular with schoolmates?
7. Is this child's overall academic performance much below average for his/her age?

The screening examination questionnaire

Eight individual tests were retained in the screening examination as follows:

1. Whistle through pouted lips
2. Make five successive skips
3. Roll tennis ball with dominant foot in spiral fashion around 6 matchboxes at 30-cm intervals
4. Throw tennis ball up, clap hands up to four times, then catch ball with both hands or with the dominant hand
5. Tie single shoelace with double bow
6. Thread 10 beads
7. Pierce 20 holes in graph paper
8. Posting box.

A detailed description of these tests is not given here as they are fully reproduced in Chapter 5 under Tests of Motor Proficiency.

When all the results of the eight screening tests on all the schoolchildren were obtained, each item was scored as a pass or fail according to the criteria developed from the pilot survey. A failure in each of the eight test items was recorded as follows:

1. Unable to whistle a musical note through pouted lips
2. Unable to make 5 successive skips after 3 attempts including, if necessary, 2 demonstrations by the examiner
3. Failure to roll the ball as required or failure to complete the test in 18 seconds
4. Failure to clap the hands more than twice before catching the tennis ball
5. Failure to tie the shoelace with a double bow or to carry out this act in less than 15 seconds
6. Failure to thread the 10 beads in less than 38 seconds
7. Failure to pierce 20 holes in graph paper in less than 24 seconds
8. Failure to insert all the posting box shapes in less than 18 seconds.

The clumsy children were selected on the following basis:

> 8-year-olds: 6 or more failures
> 9-year-olds: 5 or more failures
> 10-year-olds: 4 or more failures
> 11-year-olds: 3 or more failures
> 12-year-olds: 2 or more failures.

A clumsy child could be regarded as one in whom the Motor Standard exceeded 13 where Motor Standard = chronological age (years) + no. of screen test failures.

In order to increase the sample of clumsy children to approximately six per cent of each age group, several 'borderline' clumsy children were included amongst the subjects with the lowest motor ability to be examined neurologically and electroencephalographically. This concerned only four 8-year-olds who had scored 5 failures, five 9-year-olds who had scored 4 failures, and five 11-year-olds who had scored 2 failures. In each instance these additional 14 children were selected because they were the oldest borderline clumsy children (i.e. Motor Standard = 13) in their respective age groups. (Eventually there were altogether 56 children aged between 8 and 12 years who were deemed to be clumsy.)

Fifty-six control children were selected by matching each clumsy child with another child of the same sex who was in the same age group and same classroom. One further proviso was that the control children were not to be selected from the borderline clumsy group (i.e. Motor Standard = 13) which constituted 8-year-olds scoring 5 failures, 9-year-olds with 4 failures, 10-year-olds with 3 failures, 11-year-olds with 2 failures and 12-year-olds with 1 failure. All the other schoolchildren qualified as potential controls.

The parents of all the clumsy and control children were contacted by letter for permission to carry out the neurological and EEG examinations. Each parent was also requested to complete a questionnaire about their child. Of the 56 clumsy and 56 control children, the parents of 52 and 51 respectively approved further examination and completed questionnaires. The 95 per cent affirmative response from the parents was most heartening as it was anticipated that this would allow for greater validity in statistical analyses of the results obtained.

The questionnaire for parents

Considerable modification of the pilot survey questionnaire for parents was necessary for the improvement of data collection. Firstly, it was important to simplify the questions regarding developmental milestones as most parents were unwilling to even hazard a guess regarding the approximate time of accomplishment of some milestones. From experience gained in the pilot survey, it was found that parents were more likely to recall whether their child had achieved a particular milestone by a certain age. Thus the questions were rephrased in order to obtain either an affirmative or a negative answer, i.e. instead of asking 'At which age did your child first learn to walk without help?', this particular question was rephrased 'Did your child first learn to walk without help before aged 18 months?', answer 'yes' or 'no'. The format of the modified questionnaire for parents is given below:

STRICTLY CONFIDENTIAL

QUESTIONNAIRE FOR PARENTS

Name of child (Block letters): ....
                              Surname   First Name
Address: ....
Phone No:.............   Date:.............
Age: ....years.............months
PUT TICK IN CORRECT SPACE
Your child's ability at sporting activity is:
Above average............ Average............ Below average...............
Much below average...............
Your child's ability to use his/her hands generally is:
Above average............ Average............ Below average...............
Much below average...............
Do you think your child is *VERY* clumsy in his/her movements?
            Yes......   No......   Undecided......
Did your child first learn to:
Walk without help before aged 18 months?   Yes...... No......
Speak in sentences before aged 3 years?   Yes...... No......
Stop wetting nappies in daytime before aged 3 years? Yes...... No......
Ride tricycle before aged 4 years?   Yes...... No......
Ride bicycle before aged 8 years?   Yes...... No......
Blow nose into hanky before aged 7 years?   Yes...... No......
Use knife and fork together before aged 7 years?   Yes...... No......
Catch tennis ball from a few feet away before
    aged 8 years?   Yes...... No......
Dress for school without help for buttons and laces
    before aged 8 years?   Yes...... No......

Has your child had any of the following illnesses?

1. Unconscious from head injury   Yes . . . . . . No . . . . . .
2. Meningitis   Yes . . . . . . No . . . . . .
3. Encephalitis   Yes . . . . . . No . . . . . .
4. Convulsions with fever   Yes . . . . . . No . . . . . .
5. Any other form of convulsion, epileptic fit or seizure
   without fever   Yes . . . . . . No . . . . . .
Has your child any chronic ill heath?   Yes . . . . . . No . . . . . .
If yes, describe briefly

Father's present occupation: Mother's present occupation:
. . . .
Father's country of birth: Mother's country of birth:
. . . .
Child's country of birth: . . . .
Is your child adopted?   Yes . . . . No . . . . (if yes, do not attempt to answer any
further questions).
Father's age . . . . years   Mother's age . . . . years
List below full brothers and full sisters in order of birth:

First Name:	Age:		First Name:	Age:
1.	. . . .	6.	. . . .
2.	. . . .	7.	. . . .
3.	. . . .	8.	. . . .
4.	. . . .	9.	. . . .
5.	. . . .	10.	. . . .

Has any family member (brothers, sisters, parents, uncles, aunts, grandparents, cousins) suffered from epilepsy, fits, convulsions, mental retardation, cerebral palsy, serious mental illness, brain disease, paralysis?
Yes . . . . . . No . . . . . . If yes, state whether father, brother etc., and which disorder:
Length of pregnancy was: approximately 9 months . . . .
                          premature by more than 2 weeks . . . .
                          overdue by more than 2 weeks . . . .
                          Birth was: Normal . . . . breech . . . . forceps . . . .
caesarean . . . .
Birth weight was: $5\frac{1}{2}$ lb or more . . . . less than $5\frac{1}{2}$ lb . . . .
How many miscarriages has mother had? (loss of pregnancy before 6 months)
How many stillbirths has mother had? (pregnancy greater than 6 months)
Were there any serious problems in the first few hours, days or weeks of life?
Yes . . . . No . . . . If yes, describe briefly.

The only further modifications were deletions of relatively unimportant questions, with the desirable effect of simplifying the questionnaire.

The deleted questions pertained to:

Father's state of health
Mother's state of health
Length of labour.

Parents had difficulty in remembering accurately the length of established labour. Regarding the length of pregnancy, the parent now had the choice of three alternatives, namely, approximately 9 months, premature by more than 2 weeks, or overdue by more than 2 weeks, instead of stating the exact length of prematurity or postmaturity. Similarly, the assessment of prematurity was assisted by biasing documentation of the child's birth weight to either more or less than $5\frac{1}{2}$ lb (2500 g) in accordance with the recommendations of the WHO Expert Group on Prematurity (World Health Organisation, 1961; *Medical Journal of Australia,* 1971). Some clarification of the terms miscarriages and stillbirths seemed necessary. The former was defined as loss of pregnancy before 6 months gestation, and the latter as loss of pregnancy after 6 months.

Neurological and general examination questionnaires

The format of the questionnaire for neurological and general examination was completely unchanged and the same proforma was used as for the pilot survey in each instance and is reproduced below. The questionnaire was filled in entirely by the examiner.

NEUROLOGICAL AND GENERAL EXAMINATION

Name: .... Age:...... Sex:......
Date:.....................
Are you in good health?   Yes .... No ....
If no, explain:
Headache: .... Faints or fits: ....

Anticonvulsants: .... Menarche: ....

Sporting ability: Good or average .... Below average ....
Much below average ....
Reading age: .... years   Skull circumference .... cm
Skull contour .... Normal   Abnormal ....

Cranial nerves .... Normal   or explain abnormality

Smell
VAR
VAL
Fields
Fundi
Pupils
EOM
Nystagmus
Ptosis
Corneal reflexes
Facial CW
Facial PP
Motor V
Facial power
Hearing R
Hearing L

Palate
Swallow and Voice
Sternomastoids and Trapezii
Tongue midline
Tone: Normal .... Gen. Hypotonia .... Increased ...... Explain ....
Power: Normal ....
    UMN weakness   mild ....   mod ......   severe ....   explain ....
    LMN weakness   mild ....   mod ......   severe ....   explain ....
    Hemiplegia   Quadriplegia   Diplegia
Chorea: Nil .... Mild .... Moderate .... Severe .... Unilateral ....
Other abnormal movements: Explain
Finger/nose:
Normal .... R. abnormal .... L. abnormal .... Both abnormal ....
Rapid hand movement
Normal .... R. abnormal .... L. abnormal .... Both abnormal ....
Fine finger movement
Normal .... R. abnormal .... L. abnormal .... Both abnormal ....
Heel/knee/shin:
Normal .... R. abnormal .... L. abnormal .... Both abnormal ....
Rapid foot movement
Normal .... R. abnormal .... L. abnormal .... Both abnormal ....
Deep reflexes:
Brisk ...... sluggish ...... absent ...... hyperactive L ...... hyperactive R ....
both hyperactive .... clonus L .... clonus R .... bilat. clonus ....
Explain: ....
Plantars: Flexor .... R. ext .... L. ext .... Both ext ....
Abdominals: Normal .... Absent L .... Absent R .... All absent ....
Sensation: Normal .... Abnormal .... Explain ....
General: Normal .... Abnormal .... Explain ....
BP   Systolic .... Diastolic ....
Congenital abnormalities: Nil .... or explain ....
Speech: Normal .... mild stammer .... severe stammer ....
            mild dysarthria .... severe dysarthria ....
General inspection: Normal .... or explain ....
Co-operation: Normal .... below average .... much below average ....
Hyperactivity: Nil .... Mild .... Moderate or severe ....

At this stage a supplementary neurological examination was also included
and its first section comprised eight test items modified from the original
screening examination shown below.

SUPPLEMENTARY NEUROLOGICAL EXAMINATION—SECTION 1

Name: ....
1. Hop on dominant leg 10 times without error (3 attempts)
2. Foot dominance (hop, kick)   R   L   RL
3. Walk heel to toe along line without adjustments (3 attempts)
4. Stereognosis (8 articles hidden in bag)   .... seconds
5. Copy finger postures: 'thumb between', 'cross fingers',
                   'benediction'

6. Finger sense (dominant hand)—'in between' (2, 1, 3, 1, 0)
7. Raise your left hand
   Touch your right hand on your left ear
   Touch my left elbow with your right hand
8. Hand dominance   R   L   RL

A failure in the hopping test meant inability to hop 10 times on the preferred leg without overbalancing on to the other leg. Foot dominance was scored as 'right' if the preferred foot for hopping and kicking was the right foot, and vice versa for left dominance. If the child hopped on one foot and kicked with the other, he or she was deemed to have 'crossed dominance'. Similarly hand dominance was assessed with respect to the preferred hand for writing and for throwing a ball. If a larger number of tests of hand and foot dominance were to have been used, many more children would have qualified as 'crossed dominant' for hand or for foot, but it was expedient to compare the clumsy children with their controls for only the contingencies mentioned. All the remaining tests were precisely the same as used in the pilot survey.

The second section of the supplementary neurological examination was a modification of the pilot survey group screening examination. On this occasion the child was required only to write 'The quick brown fox jumps over the lazy dog' and the numbers 12,345 and 6079 in numerals. He was requested to draw a circle and insert the numbers 1 to 12 as in a clock-face, then insert the minute and hour hands indicating the time at 10 minutes to 2 o'clock. The rest of the quarto-sized page issued to each child was used to copy 5 geometric figures into appropriate areas as in the pilot survey.

EEG questionnaire

Finally an electroencephalogram was carried out on each of the clumsy and control children and scored on exactly the same proforma used in the pilot survey which is reproduced below.

ELECTROENCEPHALOGRAM

Name: .... Date: ....
Age: .... years .... months   Sex: M .... F ....
Medication: Nil .... or write here: ....
Urine: N.A.D. .... Sugar .... Alb ....
Excess eye artifact.   No .... Yes ....
Excess movement artifact.   No .... Yes ......
Excess muscle artifact.   No .... Yes ....
Organisation:
Normal .... Fair .... Poor ....
Dominant post. rhythm: .... Hz
Dominant ant. rhythm: .... Hz
Alpha amplitude: L .... μV
Alpha amplitude: R .... μV
Alpha blocking: Yes .... No ....

Frequencies:	symm . . . . slow L . . . . slow R . . . .
Beta:	nil . . . . L . . . . R . . . . Bil . . . .
Theta:	nil . . . . L . . . . R . . . . Bil . . . .
Excess Theta:	nil . . . . L . . . . R . . . . Bil . . . .
Delta:	nil . . . . L . . . . R . . . . Bil . . . .
Parox. Theta:	nil . . . . L . . . . R . . . . Bil . . . .
Random sharp:	nil . . . . L . . . . R . . . . Bil . . . .
Focal sharp:	nil . . . . L . . . . R . . . . Bil . . . .
Random spikes:	nil . . . . L . . . . R . . . . Bil . . . .
Focal spikes:	nil . . . . L . . . . R . . . . Bil . . . .
Paroxys. SW:	nil . . . . L . . . . R . . . . Bil . . . .
3/sec SW:	nil . . . . L . . . . R . . . . Bil . . . .
HV response:	theta: No . . . . Yes . . . .
HV response:	delta: No . . . . Yes . . . .
HV recovery:	less 1 mt . . . . more . . . .
HV sharp:	No . . . . Yes . . . .
HV spikes:	No . . . . Yes . . . .
Photic driving:	Bil . . . . L . . . . R . . . . Nil . . . .
Photic spikes:	No . . . . Yes . . . .
Photic slow waves:	No . . . . Yes . . . .
Sleep study:	No . . . . Yes . . . .
Spindles:	No . . . . L . . . . R . . . . Bil . . . .
Humps:	No . . . . L . . . . R . . . . Bil . . . .
14 and 6:	No . . . . L . . . . R . . . . Bil . . . .
Spikes:	No . . . . Yes . . . .
Spikes parox:	No . . . . R . . . . L . . . . Bil . . . .
Parox. slow:	No . . . . R . . . . L . . . . Bil . . . .
Drowsy spikes:	No . . . . R . . . . L . . . . Bil . . . .
Abnormality in record:	No . . . . Yes . . . .

IF ABNORMAL

Borderline . . . . mild . . . . mod . . . . severe . . . .
Diffuse . . . . focal . . . . bil . . . .
Epileptic features: No . . . . Yes . . . .

IF FOCAL

Bilateral	F . . . . T . . . . P . . . . O . . . .
Left	F . . . . T . . . . P . . . . O . . . . All . . . .
Right	R . . . . T . . . . P . . . . O . . . . All . . . .

Summary:

Results of the Total Definitive Survey

Age and sex distribution

The data collected from the pilot survey at WLSS were pooled with the information obtained from the other four schools comprising 992 children altogether. There were 276 children from WLSS (3 were deleted because of insufficient data) aged 6 to 12 years inclusive and 716 children from the other four schools aged 8 to 12 years inclusive. The age and sex distribution in all five schools are given in Table 4.9. The period that each child had been under his or her individual teacher's surveillance is shown in Table 4.10.

All the six- and seven-year-old children of the pilot survey are now excluded from further consideration here. Further analysis in this section is of the 919 8- to 12-year-old children in the survey.

On the basis of their inferior performance in the eight screening tests, an additional 30 clumsy children were selected from the 716 children in the four schools apart from the pilot survey. One clumsy child from the pilot survey was excluded because of incomplete data leaving 12 more from the pilot survey who still qualified as 'clumsy' for the total survey. The overall total of 56 clumsy children was obtained by including the 14 borderline clumsy subjects described earlier. Table 4.11 gives the screening test scores (i.e.

Table 4.9. Age and sex distribution of all children

Age	Sex	WLSS	LSS	PMS	CC	SH	Total	
6	M	17	0	0	0	0	17	36
	F	19	0	0	0	0	19	
7	M	16	0	0	0	0	16	37
	F	21	0	0	0	0	21	
8	M	16	21	0	24	0	61	114
	F	14	18	0	0	21	53	
9	M	28	18	0	38	0	84	144
	F	16	22	0	0	22	60	
10	M	18	27	0	44	0	89	165
	F	25	21	0	0	30	76	
11	M	24	35	1	64	0	124	191
	F	24	13	0	0	30	67	
12	M	18	14	48	97	0	177	305
	F	20	7	51	0	50	128	
Total	M	276	196	100	267	153	568	992
	F						424	

Table 4.10. Period of observation by schoolteacher

Months of observation	Number of children
0–6	752
7–12	169
13–24	43
Over 24	28
Total	992

Table 4.11. Screening test scores of clumsy children showing age and sex distribution

| | Number of failures | | | | | | | | | | | | | |
| | 2 | | 3 | | 4 | | 5 | | 6 | | 7 | | 8 | |
Age	M	F	M	F	M	F	M	F	M	F	M	F	M	F
8							3	1	3					
9					3	2	1	1			1			
10					5	2	1	1						
11	3	2	4	1	1	1								
12	5	5	3	2	3				1				1	

Table 4.12. Age and sex distribution of clumsy children

Age	Sex	Number	Percentage
8	Male	3	4.9
	Female	4	7.5
	Total	7	6.1
9	Male	4	4.8
	Female	4	6.7
	Total	8	5.6
10	Male	6	6.7
	Female	3	3.9
	Total	9	5.5
11	Male	8	6.6
	Female	4	6.0
	Total	12	6.3
12	Male	12	6.8
	Female	8	6.3
	Total	20	6.7
8–12	Male	33	6.2
	Female	23	6.0
	Total	56	6.1

number of failures out of eight tests) of the clumsy children and shows the age and sex distribution.

Table 4.12 illustrates that there was an almost equal sex incidence of clumsiness in the 8- to 12-year-old schoolchild population which was sampled.

Teachers' questionnaire

In the data obtained from both the schoolteachers and the individual screening examination, the clumsy children were compared with all the other children in the series, but in follow-up studies including neurological examination and electroencephalogram, the clumsy children were compared with their controls.

The answers to the seven principal questions below are analysed in Tables 4.13 to 4.19. The last question, 'Is this child's overall academic performance much below average for his age?', was not included in the pilot survey. For each of the questions, the answer was given as 'yes', 'no' or 'possible'.

1. Is the formation and neatness of this child's handwriting much below average? (Table 4.13)
2. Is the child's sporting ability and bodily agility much below average? (Table 4.14)
3. Is the child unduly clumsy? (Table 4.15)
4. Does the child fidget excessively in class? (Table 4.16)
5. Is the child's conduct much below average? (Table 4.17)
6. Is the child unpopular with schoolmates? (Table 4.18)
7. Is this child's overall academic performance much below average for his age? (Table 4.19).

Table 4.13. Teachers' questionnaire—poor handwriting

	Clumsy	All others	Significance
Yes	11	66	$P < 0.01$
Yes + possible	18	154	$P < 0.05$
Total	56	863	

Table 4.14. Teachers' questionnaire—low sporting ability

	Clumsy	All others	Significance
Yes	14	31	$P < 0.001$
Yes + possible	26	154	$P < 0.001$
Total	56	863	

Table 4.15. Teachers' questionnaire—clumsiness

	Clumsy	All others	Significance
Yes	8	20	$P < 0.001$
Yes + possible	22	105	$P < 0.001$
Total	56	863	

Table 4.16. Teachers' questionnaire—fidgetiness

	Clumsy	All others	Significance
Yes	11	87	$P < 0.05$
Yes + possible	17	157	$P < 0.05$
Total	56	863	

Table 4.17. Teachers' questionnaire—bad conduct

	Clumsy	All others	Significance
Yes	6	30	$P < 0.05$
Yes + possible	10	71	$P < 0.05$
Total	56	863	

Table 4.18. Teachers' questionnaire—unpopularity

	Clumsy	All others	Significance
Yes	5	13	$P < 0.001$
Yes + possible	13	82	$P < 0.001$
Total	56	863	

Table 4.19. Teachers' questionnaire—poor academic performance

	Clumsy	All others	Significance
Yes	10	54	$P < 0.001$
Yes + possible	16	117	$P < 0.01$
Total	41	675	

The eight screening tests

As the clumsy children were selected on the basis of their inferior performance in these tests, it is axiomatic that a highly significant difference between the results in the clumsy children and all the other children would occur. However, these analyses were helpful in indicating the degree of reliability of the individual tests. The actual results are not given here, but it was shown that the timed tests were clearly more reliable than the untimed tests of whistling, skipping, and throwing and catching the tennis ball.

Table 4.20. Age and sex distribution of clumsy and control children in follow-up observations

Age	Sex	Clumsy	Control
	Male	3	3
8	Female	3	4
	Total	6	7
	Male	4	4
9	Female	4	5
	Total	8	9
	Male	6	5
10	Female	3	4
	Total	9	9
	Male	8	8
11	Female	3	3
	Total	11	11
	Male	10	8
12	Female	8	7
	Total	18	15
8–12	Male	31	28
	Female	21	23
	Total	52	51

The following data illustrate the observed differences between the clumsy children and their controls. Of the 56 clumsy children and their matched controls, 52 clumsy children and 51 controls reported for follow-up. Only 46 of the clumsy children followed up therefore were perfectly matched with their own controls and the other five clumsy children and four controls were not age matched. It was considered justifiable to analyse the combined results of all the 103 clumsy and control children followed up as most of the observations were not age dependent.

Table 4.20 shows the age and sex distribution of the clumsy children and control children in the follow-up survey.

Parents' questionnaire

The information obtained from the parents of the clumsy children and the controls is contained in Tables 4.21 to 4.29.

There was no difference between the clumsy children and their controls with regard to father's or mother's occupation and country of birth, or the child's country of birth.

The tendency for a higher incidence of firstborn in clumsy children (Table 4.28) was reflected in their lower parental age.

A positive family history of neurological illness or any specific abnormal perinatal factor was not forthcoming.

Table 4.21. Parents' questionnaire—ability at sport

Category	Clumsy	Control	Significance
Above average	5	5	N.S.
Average	34	44	N.S.
Below average	7	0	N.S.
Much below average	5	0	N.S.
Below and Much below average	12	0	$P < 0.001$

Table 4.22. Parents' questionnaire—ability to use hands

Category	Clumsy	Control	Significance
Above average	5	7	N.S.
Average	39	43	N.S.
Below average	6	1	N.S.
Much below average	0	0	N.S.
Below and Much below average	6	1	N.S.

Table 4.23. Parents' questionnaire—very clumsy movements

Category	Clumsy	Control	Significance
No	42	48	N.S.
Yes	5	3	N.S.
Yes and Undecided	8	3	N.S.

Table 4.24. Parents' questionnaire—developmental achievements

Question		Clumsy		Control		Significance
	Before	Yes	No	Yes	No	
Walk	18 months	46	6	48	3	N.S.
Speech	3 years	40	10	46	5	N.S.
Dry	3 years	43	9	49	2	N.S.
Tricycle	4 years	40	12	47	4	N.S.
Bicycle	8 years	30	22	36	14	N.S.
Blow nose	7 years	45	7	50	0	$P < 0.05$
Cutlery	7 years	44	7	43	8	N.S.
Catch ball	8 years	39	12	47	2	$P < 0.05$
Dressing	8 years	35	16	48	2	$P < 0.001$

Table 4.25. Parents' questionnaire—past history

Question	Clumsy		Control		Significance
	Yes	No	Yes	No	
Concussion	2	49	2	49	N.S.
Meningitis	1	51	0	51	N.S.
Encephalitis	0	52	0	50	N.S.
Febrile fits	2	50	3	48	N.S.
Epilepsy	1	51	0	51	N.S.
Chronic illness	12	40	9	42	N.S.

Table 4.26. Parents' questionnaire—adopted children

Adopted	Clumsy	Control	Significance
Yes	4	0	N.S.
No	48	51	N.S.

Table 4.27. Parents' questionnaire—average ages of parents on child's birthday

Parent	Clumsy	Control
Fathers	34	37
Mothers	28	32

Table 4.28. Parents' questionnaire—birth rank

Rank	Clumsy	Control
Firstborn	20	11
Second	16	15
Third	7	12
Fourth	5	9
Fifth	2	3
Sixth or more	2	1

Table 4.29. Parents' questionnaire—number in sibship

Sibship	Clumsy	Control
1	5	2
2	13	11
3	12	16
4	8	13
5	5	6
6	5	2
6+	4	1

Not significant

Neurological and general examination

No differences were found on specific interrogation of the clumsy children as opposed to their controls except with regard to the child's own assessment of his or her sporting ability (Table 4.30).

The clumsy children tended to have lower reading quotients and intelligence quotients than their controls (Tables 4.31 and 4.32).

On physical examination there was no difference in height and weight between the two groups and no child had an abnormally large or small head circumference. The rest of the physical findings are summarised in Tables 4.33 to 4.36.

Table 4.30. Sporting ability (child's own assessment)

Classification	Clumsy	Control	Significance
Good or Average	33	47	$P < 0.01$
Below average	9	4	Not significant
Much below average	10	0	$P < 0.01$
Below and Much below average	19	4	$P < 0.001$

Table 4.31. Reading quotient

	Clumsy	Control	Significance
Mean RQ	96	107	
RQ < 80	12	3	$P < 0.05$
80–99	20	15	
100–119	13	20	
120 and over	7	14	

Table 4.32. Intelligence quotient

	Clumsy	Control	Significance
Mean IQ	98	111	
IQ < 80	10	0	$P < 0.01$
80–99	14	10	
100–119	20	27	
120 and over	8	15	

Table 4.33. Cranial nerves—abnormal findings

Physical sign	Clumsy	Control
(Total examined)	(52)	(51)
Anosmia	0	0
Visual acuity less than 6/9		
Right (uncorrected)	1	1
Left (uncorrected)	3	0
Abnormal visual fields on confrontation	0	0
Abnormal optic fundi	0	0
Abnormal pupils	0	0
External ocular palsy	1	0
Nystagmus	1	0
Ptosis	0	0
Absent corneal reflex	0	0
Facial anaesthesia	0	0
Weak muscles of mastication	0	0
Facial weakness	0	0
Deafness (Right)	1	1
(Left)	2	1
Palatal weakness	0	0
Dysphagia and dysphonia	0	0
Sternomastoid and trapezius weakness	0	0
Lingual weakness	0	0

Table 4.34. Motor system—abnormal findings

Physical sign	Clumsy	Control
Hypotonia	2	1
Spasticity	0	0
Weakness of a limb, hemiplegia or diplegia	0	0
Mild chorea (chorea minima)	12	2
Moderate chorea	1	0
Other abnormal movements (i.e. tic)	1	0
Abnormal finger-nose test	0	0
Abnormal rapid hand movement	0	0
Abnormal fine finger movement	3	0
Abnormal heel-knee-shin test	2	0
Abnormal rapid foot movement	0	0
Absent deep tendon reflexes	1	0
Asymmetrical deep tendon reflexes	1	0
Hyperactive deep tendon reflexes	0	1
Bilateral Babinski sign	1	0
Unilateral Babinski sign'	1	0
Absent abdominal reflexes	0	0

Table 4.35. Further physical examination—abnormal findings

Physical sign	Clumsy	Control
Sensation	1	1
General examination (abnormal findings)	5	1
Congenital abnormalities on inspection	1	1
Severe stammer	1	1
Severe dysarthria (developmental)	0	1
Mild dysarthria (developmental)	3	0
Abnormal general inspection	1	0
Poor co-operation	0	0
Mild hyperactivity	2	0

There were no significant differences in the findings on general examination.

Table 4.36. Summary of neurological abnormalities

(A) Clumsy children
Case No.
    (1) Mild chorea; impaired fine finger movements, absent deep tendon reflexes, impaired vibration sense in fingers and toes
    (2) General slowness of movement
    (5) Mild chorea
    (6) Mild generalised hypotonia
    (9) Generalised hypotonia
    (16) Unequal deep tendon reflexes, extensor plantar
    (24) Moderate chorea
    (25) Mild chorea
    (30) Mild chorea
    (31) Mild chorea
    (33) General slowness of movement
    (35) Mild chorea
    (39) Mild chorea
    (40) Mild chorea
    (42) Mild dysarthria, apraxic attempts with fine finger movements and heel-knee-shin test
    (43) Mild dysarthria
    (46) Mild chorea, apraxic heel-knee-shin tests, extensor plantars
    (47) Mild chorea
    (50) Left external rectus palsy, nystagmus right lateral gaze, severe stammer
    (51) Mild chorea
    (52) Apraxic fine finger movement, shortened tendo Achilles, mild dyslalia

(B) Control children
    (4) Impaired vibration sense and two point discrimination in fingers
    (13) Mild chorea
    (18) Hyperactive deep tendon reflexes
    (33) Nystagmoid eye movements in primary position

Thus there were 21 clumsy children and 4 controls with neurological signs ($P < 0.001$), and 12 clumsy children and 1 control with chorea ($P < 0.001$).

Supplementary neurological examination

There was an unexpected lack of clear differentiation in the performance between clumsy and control children in tests for hopping, and walking heel to toe. Stereognosis, copying finger postures, finger sense and right–left orientation were carried out better by the control children than by the clumsy children, but in no instance did the differences reach statistical significance. The results of the determinations for cerebral dominance are interesting as there were many more clumsy children than control children with crossed dominance, but once again these results did not reach statistical significance (Table 4.37).

Again the clumsy children had poorer handwriting, topographical orientation and spatial sense than their controls, but in general the differences observed were not great.

Table 4.37. Supplementary examination—hand and foot dominance (all age groups collectively)

Dominance	Clumsy	Control
Right-handed and right-footed	27	31
Left-handed and left-footed	2	6
Concordant dominance (right or left)	29	37
Crossed dominance	23	14
Not significant		

Table 4.38. EEG—organisation of record

Organisation	Clumsy	Control
Normal	28	38
Fair	22	10
Poor	2	3
Not significant		

Electroencephalograms

All age groups were considered collectively with regard to the electroencephalographic observations. The clumsy children did not have a greater amount of artifact in their recordings. They did, however, tend to have poorer organisation of their records (Table 4.38) and a broader spectrum of dominant posterior electroencephalographic rhythms (Table 4.39). There was no greater tendency to alpha blockade with eye opening and only one of the clumsy children and no controls had significant asymmetry in the tracing.

Table 4.40 gives an analysis of the normal and abnormal EEG rhythms.

Table 4.39. EEG—dominant posterior rhythm

Frequency (Hz)	Clumsy	Control
< 8	2	0
8	4	9
9	8	13
10	25	21
11	8	5
12	4	1
13	1	1
>13	0	1
	Not significant	

Table 4.40. EEG—Normal and abnormal rhythms

Rhythm	Category	Nil	Unilateral	Bilateral
Beta	Clumsy	11	0	41
	Control	11	1	39
Theta	Clumsy	5	0	47
	Control	8	1	42
Excess theta	Clumsy	40	1	11
	Control	48	0	3
Delta	Clumsy	51	1	0
	Control	51	0	0
Paroxysmal theta	Clumsy	45	1	6
	Control	48	0	3
Paroxysmal delta	Clumsy	51	1	0
	Control	51	0	0
Random sharp	Clumsy	34	1	17
	Control	45	0	6
Focal sharp	Clumsy	48	3	1
	Control	49	1	0
Focal spikes	Clumsy	50	2	0
	Control	49	2	0
Random spikes	Clumsy	51	0	1
	Control	50	0	1
Paroxysmal spike-wave	Clumsy	49	0	3
	Control	49	1	1
3 per second spike-wave	Clumsy	52	0	0
	Control	51	0	0

There were no significant differences in the responses in the two groups to the effect of hyperventilation, but better bilateral recruiting responses were observed with photic stimulation in the controls. As sleep studies were carried out on only 4 clumsy children and 3 control children, they were not considered for further analysis. Ten clumsy children and 4 control children had electroencephalograms which exhibited spikes or paroxysmal features. There was no significant region in which focal abnormalities appeared in the electroencephalograms of the clumsy children. The total number of EEG abnormalities and a further analysis of the types of abnormalities are given in Tables 4.41 and 4.42.

Table 4.41. EEG—total number of abnormal records

Degree of abnormality	Clumsy	Control	Significance
Normal	29	42	
Borderline	6	2	
Mild	14	5	
Moderate	3	2	
Severe	0	0	
Total abnormal	23	9	$P < 0.01$

Reproduced with the kind permission of the editors of *Proceedings of the Australian Association of Neurologists* and *The Medical Journal of Australia*.

Table 4.42. EEG—types of abnormalities

Type of abnormality	Clumsy (23)	Control (9)
Epileptogenic features	10	4
Diffuse abnormality	13	4
Focal abnormality	4	2
Bilateral abnormality	6	3

Reproduced with the kind permission of the editors of *Proceedings of the Australian Association of Neurologists* and *The Medical Journal of Australia*.

Normative Data and Final Standardisation of Screening Tests

This section collates data obtained from the screening tests of motor ability carried out on all 992 children in the total survey including the pilot survey. Only the values obtained from the 8- to 12-year-old children could be standardised satisfactorily as there were insufficient numbers of six- and seven-year-olds who had now been excluded from further study after the completion of the pilot survey. The 5th, 10th, 50th, 90th and 95th percentile levels of proficiency in the remaining five timed tests were computed and expressed numerically in seconds time. The remaining three tests were computed on a pass-fail basis within these percentile ratings. From the values obtained, a child's scores in the eight tests of motor proficiency can be readily converted into percentile estimations. It is suggested that if a child were to score below the 10th percentile for his age group in only one test, the result might be spurious and probably of no significance, two scores below the 10th percentile might be of borderline significance, whereas three or more scores below the 10th percentile should be regarded as significant. The degree of clumsiness could also be estimated according to the total scores below 10th or 5th percentiles.

The complete proforma of the eight screening tests including the method of scoring and all relevant percentile tables are given in Chapter 5.

SUMMARY AND CONCLUSIONS

The Pilot Survey

The aim of the pilot survey was to make a trial of screening tests of motor performance on the pupils of one primary school. The children with performance levels in the lowest 10 per cent of the range of each age were selected for further neurological assessment and EEG. It was felt that the standardisation of these tests after the pilot survey would permit the rapid selection of other children from the total survey who were within the lowest range of manual dexterity and bodily agility. The defects in the general organisation of the pilot survey were also modified to allow for a smoother operation of the total survey. The principles involved in obtaining the children with the poorest motor performance and matching them with controls of the same age and sex in the same classroom were described.

The test results comprising the selection of the clumsy children and their controls were explained. Correlations were then made between the initial observations by the schoolteachers and the screening examination on the 19 clumsy children and their 19 controls. There was a very good agreement between the schoolteachers' observations on the individual children in this group and the observations borne out by the screening examinations. There was an obvious dichotomy between the results of the screening examinations on the clumsy children and their controls as anticipated because these children were actually selected on the basis of their performance in the screening examinations.

The next section dealt with the comparison of follow-up observations on 17 clumsy children and 18 controls. The results showed a definite trend towards poorer performance by the clumsy children according to data obtained from the parents' questionnaires and neurological examination. Electro-encephalographically the clumsy children had significantly more abnormalities than their controls ($P < 0.05$). The standardised screening tests were not only used for the criteria of selection of clumsy children in the rest of the total survey, but also were applied retrospectively to the children in the pilot survey. The children so selected by these modified criteria were added to those selected with the rest of the definitive total survey for further analysis.

One of the more important aspects of this preliminary investigation was the

validation of the eight tests used to select clumsy children on the basis of
confirmatory evidence by the parents, teachers and schoolchildren. Thus the
clumsy children selected through the criteria of the screening examinations had
a significantly higher incidence of motor problems reported either by
themselves, their schoolteachers or their parents than the control children
($P < 0.01$). This confirmation of the validity of the devised screening tests
justified their further employment in the total survey. The standardised eight
screening test results have been given in Table 4.6 where the lower limit of
normal performance is shown. It was recognised that the test standards would
need revision after the completion of the total survey.

The Definitive Total Survey

Thirty-three per cent more boys than girls participated in the total survey.
This bias in sex distribution was due to the larger population of 8- to 12-year-
olds in the private boys' school than in the private girls' school and is also
evident from Table 4.9 in each of the other age groups. The great majority of
the children had been under the individual schoolteacher's surveillance for five
months or more as the tests were never administered before the sixth month of
an academic year.

From the time of the pilot survey it was evident that the screening tests
devised were unsuitable for six- and seven-year-olds who therefore were
deleted from the total survey. Data regarding these children are not presented,
as they could be only accepted as an approximate assessment.

The apparent equal sex incidence of clumsy children in the population
sample might be misleading because the clumsiest children in the entire
population probably had been excluded from most ordinary schools. It is
probable that a male preponderance does in fact exist as in most
developmental neurological afflictions such as developmental dyslexia.

Significant differences between the performance of the clumsy children and
all the other children were noted by their schoolteachers in each of the seven
questionnaire categories. The differences were highly significant regarding
sporting ability and clumsiness and validate the screening test selection of the
clumsy children. Interestingly, the differences regarding handwriting were less
significant, probably because there are other important factors concerned in
the formulation and neatness of an individual's handwriting apart from
adroitness of hand control. The excessive fidgetiness of the clumsy children
confirms the observations made in Chapter 2, which in turn refer to similar
conclusions made by Prechtl and Stemmer (1962). The propensity towards
frustration in clumsy children must have increased the tendency to disturbed
behaviour patterns with misconduct in the classroom (Table 4.17) and, more
importantly, towards exclusion by their peers as relative social outcasts
(Table 4.18).

The generally high degree of differentiation between clumsy children and all
other children in their performance in the screening tests is axiomatic as the
clumsy children were selected on the basis of their incompetence in these tests.
However, the results indicated a varying degree of reliability of each test. Thus,

tests 3, 6, 7 and 8 all exhibited highly significant differences in all age groups ($P < 0.001$). In each of the four other tests, the best correlations between the individual results and overall clumsiness were amongst the older age groups.

The information obtained from the completed parents' questionnaires was less reliable because the parents would naturally have shown more bias towards their children than the more objective assessments of their schoolteachers or the totally objective screening tests. Nevertheless, the results did show a definite trend towards superior performance and development in the control children. Even the parents recognised a highly significant inferior performance in the sporting abilities of the clumsy children group. The most significant retarded developmental milestones included: (1) blowing the nose into a handkerchief; (2) catching a tennis ball from a few feet away; and (3) dressing for school. The last was the most highly significant and corresponds well to earlier observations regarding dressing apraxia in these children.

No real correlation could be seen between a child's clumsiness and past history of neurological or other illness including concussion, meningitis, encephalitis, or fits; or a family history of neurological disease. There was also no real correlation with the following factors:

1. Father's or mother's occupation
2. Father's, mother's or child's country of birth
3. Adoption.

It can be seen from Table 4.27 that the parents of the clumsy children tended to be younger than the parents of the control children. This is readily explicable by the greater proportion (38 per cent) of clumsy children who were first-born as opposed to their controls (21 per cent). The total size of the sibship was of no consequence.

Prematurity, postmaturity, abnormal delivery and neonatal illness were not commoner in the clumsy group, neither was there a higher incidence of sibling death in utero. Even an analysis of the composite of (1) a history of past neurological illness and (2) all abnormal perinatal factors failed to disclose significant differences between the two groups.

The results of follow-up interrogation and physical assessment including neurological examination yielded some important significant data. Just as their schoolteachers and their parents had recognised a significant ineptitude in their sporting ability, the clumsy children themselves had insight into their inadequacy in this regard ($P < 0.001$). There were less significant differences in reading ability and overall general intelligence, but no differences in bodily configuration including height, weight and head circumference.

In the neurological physical examination there were no obvious consistent features in the clumsy children apart from the increased manifestation of choreiform movements ($P < 0.01$). If these movements were to be accepted as a physical sign indicating neurological dysfunction, then 40 per cent of clumsy children as opposed to 8 per cent of the controls manifested neurological signs including choreiform movements ($P < 0.001$).

None of the tests in the supplementary neurological examination were of good discriminatory value although doubtless, if they were to be applied to children manifesting severer degrees of clumsiness, they would elicit significant differences. The pilot survey had already demonstrated the limited value of these tests in mildly afflicted children. Although there were more left-handed, left-footed controls than clumsy children, 44 per cent of the clumsy children manifested crossed dominance whereas only 27 per cent of the controls were in this category. This observation supports the suggestion that some of the manifestations of developmental apraxia are due to a confusion in cerebral dominance.

Other data not shown suggested a higher incidence of developmental dyslexia in clumsy children, but one which did not reach statistical significance. Again, the performance in tests for topographical sense and constructional praxis was not significantly lower although the clumsiest children did show disabilities in this regard.

The general configuration of the electroencephalograms was analysed in detail, but there were no obvious characteristics. However, there were many more unspecified abnormalities in the recordings of the clumsy children, in that 44 per cent of the clumsy children and 17 per cent of the controls had abnormal tracings ($P < 0.01$). The 17 per cent of abnormal tracings amongst the controls is consistent with the 22 per cent incidence of abnormal tracings (including borderline abnormal) amongst controls in a separate study on autistic children by the same observers (Gubbay, Lobascher and Kingerlee, 1970a, b; Lobascher, Kingerlee and Gubbay, 1970). Diffuse rather than focal EEG abnormality was commoner, although there was a higher incidence of dysrhythmia amongst the clumsy children. On this occasion the EEG recordist did not confirm an increased incidence of artifact in the tracings as had previously been reported in Chapter 3 and also by Prechtl and Stemmer (1962).

Tests of Motor Proficiency

Standardised tests of motor performance may have two principal uses. Firstly, they can be employed in the objective assessment of a particular child's motor aptitude and provide an accurate basis for comparison with children of the same age group. Secondly, the tests can be administered to large groups of children for screening purposes and expedite the identification of individuals with specific motor problems. It must be a common experience for all paediatricians to encounter over-anxious parents who are unduly worried by their child's motor ineptitude. For such parents, standardised assessment showing little deviation from the average could provide reassurance. On the other hand, even if the problem of clumsiness were to be irrefutably present, it could be of great assistance for all concerned to have some idea of the deviation from the norm. Screening tests on large numbers of subjects have the main virtue of providing an early identification of inept children who otherwise might have developed secondary problems because of lack of appreciation and understanding by teachers or parents. Even if no specific treatment could or should be instituted for a clumsy child, the early identification could provide some prophylaxis against secondary emotional problems.

Yates (1966) points out that tests of brain damage serve no useful purpose if they can identify factors only in cases where brain damage is obvious—for example in a routine neurological examination. A neurologist is in a favourable situation to design these tests because he can appreciate how certain neurological signs would take precedence in the assessment of cerebral dysfunction. Educational psychologists are highly sophisticated in the administration and interpretation of tests of motor ability and it would be inappropriate, if not improper, for any untrained person to administer or interpret their tests. There is a definite need, however, for tests of motor ability which can be administered effectively by medical and other professional personnel who have not been trained to the degree of expertise possessed by clinical psychologists. Just as standardised reading tests could be administered by the physician with ease, so should he also be able to evaluate other matters of educational importance, because it is the physician who is often the professional person to whom parents will first go for advice (Eisenberg, 1959).

Standards of normal for motor achievement such as tying shoelaces are not well established (Paine and Oppé, 1966). Stott (1966) has discussed the development of tests of motor impairment and has proposed a number of criteria which should be applied for test items before they can be regarded as satisfactory. It is unlikely that any would satisfy the more important criteria which apply to the eight screening tests described in Chapter 5 as follows:

1. They can be carried out efficiently by a person of professional status after reading the instructions or observing a demonstration.
2. They take less than 5 minutes even if administered to a subject with particular ineptitude.
3. They have been shown to identify children who have a high incidence of encephalopathy and who exhibit a very high incidence of failure of motor performance according to the more subjective assessment of their teachers and their parents.
4. There is ready access to simplified normative data.

Such tests of course should never be considered in isolation and no firm conclusions should ever be drawn from them, but they should be used only as useful guides in diagnostic orientation. Many valuable tests have already been developed, but these presuppose a certain degree of expertise by the tester. These tests have been evolved and described by the following authors: Da Costa (Ozeretzky) (1946), Elizur (1959), Ayres (1964a, b, 1966), Bergès and Lézine (1965), Bergèes (1966), Zausmer and Tower (1966), Brenner and Gillman (1966, 1968), Benton (1968), Ozer and Richardson (1969), Rabe (1969), Stott, Moyes and Headridge (1970), Touwen and Prechtl (1970) and Frostig (1971).

Screening of Children

The N & SDCP Monograph entitled *Minimal Brain Dysfunction in Children; Educational, Medical and Health Related Services; Phase Two of a Three-Phase Project* (Haring, 1969), outlined the programme and resources which would have to be developed to provide for the needs of these children.

The following tests have been listed as useful in identification and evaluation of learning disorders:

1. Intelligence tests
    (a) Global
    (b) Verbal and/or vocabulary
    (c) Visuomotor (performance)
2. Perceptive tests—visuomotor
3. Academic achievement and diagnostic tests
    (a) Reading
    (b) Spelling and arithmetic
4. Diagnostic language tests
5. Screening and readiness tests
6. Social competence tests.

A fully co-ordinated study of any one particular child in a competent setting where these tests are utilised could be of immense value, but these tests are very time-consuming and must be applied selectively.

There is agreement on the need to examine all children who enter a school (*British Medical Journal,* 1970). The examination should be a comprehensive medical assessment and should include developmental and neurological screening tests to determine the child's mental development as well as a full physical examination. There are at present few standardised screening tests which are applied to all children. Selective examinations and the use of developmental technique require more medical time than did periodic medical inspection. Bax and Whitmore (1973) investigated the practicability and value of including in the school entrant examination a short battery of neurodevelopmental tests. The time required for these tests was treble that usually allocated. Twitchell et al (1966) drew attention to the need for the extension of routine neurological assessment to detect motor deficits. Paine (1968) remarked that most children with minimal cerebral dysfunction came to medical attention only when they were brought to light by the demands of the educational system. It is reasonable to think that their school careers would be made easier and their emotional health protected by earlier recognition.

Bateman and Schiefelbusch (1969) had little doubt that within a few years it would be possible to identify accurately a substantial proportion of those five-year-olds who, in the absence of intervention, would fully qualify later as children having learning disabilities. The principle of screening tests could be carried too far; firstly, because initial enthusiasm might lead to over-diagnosis and unnecessary selection of children for special management when their problems might have resolved with maturation alone; and secondly, as has been pointed out, the incidence of learning disabilities is sure to rise with increased use of screening measures and might lead to a point of diminishing returns in the identification of subtle learning problems. As there is still an inherent un-reliability of present methods of assessment (Wenar, 1963), it would be unwise to employ on a mass scale such tests as evolved by Ozer (1968) on the neurological evaluation of school age children until follow-up study establishes the predictive value of certain tests and allows the elimination of less predictive items.

Recommendation

Presumably some children with severe developmental apraxia are excluded from normal schools and the comparative observations between clumsy children and their controls in this study may not have highlighted some important characteristics or factors in aetiology. The survey has shown that a significant number of apparently normal children attending ordinary schools have problems which are related to inefficient motor function. The most important product of this work has been a short test battery of motor proficiency which should be employable by any person of professional standing involved in the assessment of children. This test battery has been fully standardised and evaluated and has proved to be dependable in the accurate identification of children with significant motor problems and with a much higher proportion of regular neurological signs and electroencephalographic abnormalities than found in the general juvenile population.

It is suggested that these standardised tests of motor aptitude should be used by general practitioners, paediatricians, paediatric neurologists, and school medical officers as a an adjunct to routine neurological examination. They are not intended to replace sophisticated psychological tests which should be carried out by individuals specially instructed in their use, but they offer the medical practitioner and specialist schoolteacher a new, efficient means of objective assessment of motor proficiency as a rapid office procedure. The complete proforma of these tests, including the method of scoring, is given in Chapter 5.

CHAPTER FIVE

The Assessment of the Clumsy Child

The public at large and schoolteachers in particular have become increasingly aware of the nature and significance of neurodevelopmental dysfunctions in children. Previously, problems of learning, behaviour and physical performance had been more readily accepted as individual variations in children. Both advantageous and disadvantageous characteristics were largely regarded as innate and sometimes immutable variables of ordinary children. In terms of their educational management there was a tendency for children to be graded according to their overall ability.

With a continuing improvement in quality of basic human necessities, including nutrition and health, governments have taken a greater interest in education. As a direct consequence there has been a general improvement in educational standards, but more importantly a much greater interest in the assessment of children as individuals, particularly at primary school level. Instead of a broad general grading of children according to their academic or physical ability, there has been an increasing tendency to individualised assessments. Obviously, the outcome of these more detailed assessments has been the recognition of specific factors which have had a general retarding effect on school performance. Sometimes the education of the child has been profoundly disturbed, particularly when there has been a lack of provision for such problems as specific dyslexia. One can only feel compassion for the extremely self-effacing young man who is described as 'simple' by his family or protective employer because his lack of ability to read and write has been mis-interpreted as mental backwardness. For the clumsy child, the problems may be quite comparable to those of the dyslexic child in childhood. Fortunately, in a practical sense, specific clumsiness is more specific to childhood than specific dyslexia. Compensatory mechanisms are more easily deployed by the clumsy adult than the dyslexic adult mainly because of the wider range of employment opportunities which are available to the former than to the latter.

146

With the increasing educational aspirations for children, parents and schoolteachers alike have been more anxious to recruit the assistance of all professional disciplines concerned in the assessment and management of children. They have also realised that the final common factor which differentiates one child from another is his or her cerebral function and in this context any learning ineptitude must always raise the possibility of a neurological cause. At present it is not sufficiently realised that there are usually no neuropathological implications and the variations in most instances are of a neurophysiological nature. Because of these considerations there has been a burgeoning referral rate of children with school failure for medical assessment.

The general practitioner, limited in the time that he can apportion to individual assessment of his patients, cannot develop sufficient expertise to sort out these problems with confidence. Usually, he looks to the specialist to evaluate the situation, sometimes against his better medical judgement, in the face of mounting pressure from parents and educationists. Paediatricians, paediatric neurologists and neurologists must accept at present the role of medical advisor in many instances. There is no real short cut to the lengthy, stereotyped interviews, examinations and individual explanations that are required. Unless an alternative solution is found, these specialist groups may find that their skills might not be profitably utilised in clinical problems requiring perhaps greater diagnostic judgement. However, the need for medical assessment in a very large number of children cannot be denied. An obvious solution might be the employment of a greater workforce within school medical services, where the medical practitioner serves as part of a co-ordinated team in the assessment and management of learning problems. An essential prerequisite of personnel making this type of assessment is the ability to carry out a full neurological examination with competence. It is also mandatory that a parent should accompany the child at the time of such a school medical examination which includes a full neurological appraisal of the child.

This proposition does not apply to the medical practitioner who might be retained by a school for the health care of its pupils. Such an individual needs to be competent in the field of general practice in contradistinction to the type of school medical officer who might specialise in screening children for visual, hearing and cardiac defects, etc., and to whom children are referred for neurological assessment and further counselling. The child with developmental clumsiness is within this category. Liaison with the school authorities including the headmaster or specialist schoolteacher is more likely to be facilitated than in the case of doctors working outside the school and attempting to discuss matters with sundry members of school staffs with varying degrees of success.

The principles which guide the medical practitioner in the assessment of the clumsy child are no different from those of any other basically neurological question. A suggested format of medical assessment is provided below with particular reference to specific problems encountered with clumsy children, and children with minimal cerebral dysfunction or specific learning disabilities in general.

THE MEDICAL EXAMINATION

History

In noting a stereotyped history on a printed proforma, there is a danger that detail might result in elusiveness of the major problem in hand. The experienced clinician can usually judge best for himself whether the child should be present during the interview with the parent. In general the older subject requires more reassurance than the younger and should be included in the general interview for as great a proportion of the time as possible. The wiser parent will quickly sense the opportunity for discussing more delicate matters whilst the child is dressing or undressing in a separate room.

The history taking is discussed in the eight sections which follow.

Chief symptoms and general history relating to motor skills

After explaining the reason for the interview and examination, the parent should be encouraged to talk spontaneously for as long as he or she requires. In general, little prompting is needed, and it is during this time that the doctor can orient himself in the matter of physical assessment with the view to final explanation and reassurance if possible. A proforma relating to many individual items is to be discouraged during this particular part of the history taking. Although proformas are essential in screening examinations, they do not have sufficient elasticity to allow for all contingencies in individualised assessments.

Usually the parent of the clumsy child will explain how he or she had been generally slow in the acquisition of physical skills. At a critical stage of development, usually after learning to walk, the parent might have noticed an increasing tendency to bump into objects. The problem usually comes into focus shortly after the commencement of school. The parents often become anxious when a year or two of primary school seems to result in an even wider disparity between the abilities of the child and his or her peers. Often the stresses on the child do not seem to be as prominent as those on the parents. There may be associated features of hyperactivity and behaviour disorder—even truancy in order to avoid unpleasant experiences relating to the requirements of sporting activities. Almost invariably these days, the parent will admit to being anxious about 'brain damage', a concept which might have been introduced by a 'well-meaning' individual.

Family history

Although there is likely to be a higher incidence of developmental clumsiness and related disorders in parents and siblings, the implications for obtaining a full family history are rather more devious than this. So frequently, by chance alone, there may be an incidental family history of mental backwardness, epilepsy or frank neurological disease in first- or second-degree relatives. Much reassurance might be required in these fortuitous circumstances. Conversely, there may be individuals with superior physical skills within the family. Against this more competitive background, a mildly clumsy child might be dismissed as totally inept by his relatives. In fact the consultation might well be motivated by this very factor where the aspirations of ambitious parents have been thwarted. A sound knowledge of the genetic aspects of neurological disease which can be explained in simple statistical terms is a distinct advantage to the medical advisor. Parental, especially maternal, age and also birth rank may eventually emerge as important factors relating to aetiology in developmental clumsiness. Sibling miscarriages, stillbirths and neonatal deaths may provide some clue in patients with a progressive neurological disorder.

Perinatal history

All congenital abnormalities must be assessed against a background of abnormal factors operating during pregnancy. Drug ingestion and rubella are now well recognised for their teratogenetic potential. It may be as well to enquire into the possibility of maternal diabetes, diagnostic irradiation, and evidence of pre-eclamptic toxaemia or even mundane infections of the respiratory and gastrointestinal tracts. Other infective processes which may result in intra-uterine changes of widely varying degree include syphilis, toxoplasmosis and cytomegalic inclusion body disease. The period of gestation is no less important than other considerations.

The circumstances of delivery are often described in detail by the mother who may not appreciate the extent of the normal trauma of birth processes. In the eyes of parents the most critical period of life is the process of parturition. Any hint of deviation from normal delivery such as breech, forceps or caesarean, possibly following upon prolonged labour, is likely to be perpetually blameworthy even by the most enlightened. Doctors have a real responsibility in playing down these factors by bringing them into their proper perspective.

The neonatal condition of the child, including birth weight, jaundice, feeding and all factors relating to a low Apgar rating, is of prime interest.

Developmental history

The times of the acquisition of motor milestones, especially turning to and from supine and prone positions, sitting, crawling and walking are of special relevance. A general delay of milestones would not be surprising in developmental clumsiness, whereas an early acquisition of motor skills would be unusual and should alert the examiner to the supervention of an insidiously progressive neurological condition. The most reliable single motor milestone is the time of walking independently, but of course this must not be taken out of context.

The social development of the child from the appearance of smiling to the acquisition of urinary continence and acceptable behaviour patterns is not likely to lag behind general development except in cases of mental deficiency. One cannot rely entirely upon the time of the acquisition of speech as a yardstick of intellectual development, although it may be the most useful single guide. In developmental apraxia, there may be associated developmental dysarthria including articulatory apraxia which can result in a late acquisition of motor speech. In these circumstances the early understanding of speech and response to command should be intact.

Special attention should be paid to any delay in the tendency to climb on furniture and to negotiate doorknobs and door handles. The times of acquisition of skills such as riding a tricycle and bicycle should be added to detailed enquiry into the times that a child could effectively use cutlery. The examiner should have a sufficient grasp of the developmental timetable with a good working knowledge of a few reliable indices. Children, for example, should be able to blow the nose into a handkerchief by the age of seven years and to catch a tennis ball from a few feet away, and dress and undress including buttons, bows and shoelaces by the age of eight years.

Past history

All medical disorders in the past history should be elicited, but special enquiry must be made into the possibility of head injury, meningitis, encephalitis, febrile convulsions and epilepsy. Often chronic illness such as asthma might be overlooked and prolonged hospitalisation or other institutional care may have a deleterious effect on child development. A history of behavioural problems in the past should also be sought specifically.

Social history

Often the father's or mother's occupation provides the background of parental aspiration. The experience in Newcastle upon Tyne in England was that a much larger proportion of clumsy children were referred from families with professional backgrounds. This might have given the spurious impression that developmental apraxia is more common in children of parents with high intellectual achievement, but the more logical conclusion is the disparity between background and general motor abilities. Factors of more dubious significance might be the country of origin of parents or child, whether the child is adopted, and whether there are any internal family problems relating to the household such as undue financial pressures or marital disharmony.

Psychiatric history

One of the greatest responsibilities of the medical advisor is to preserve the psychological wellbeing of the child. The role of therapist or schoolteacher may be far more important than that of the paediatrician or neurologist in this situation, but the physician has greater access to psychiatric assessment and management. It is always difficult to differentiate primary and secondary factors in the interrelationship between behaviour disorders and physical ineptitudes or learning disabilities. Even in situations where hyperactivity, negativism, anxiety and depression might be reactive factors to an unpleasant situation for the child, an easing of the mental burden might have a salutary effect on performance because of an improvement in attention span and concentration in general.

School history

The child's performance at school is fundamental to the whole issue and the most obvious factor is whether the child's grade is appropriate to his chronological age. His attitude to the schoolteacher and to his class conditions his achievement level. Often the specific problems of a child in either the academic or sporting spheres may be borne out by specific interrogation relating to matters involving the school history. An important adjunct to obtaining information from both child and parent is liaison with the headmaster, specialist schoolteacher or class teacher after obtaining parental approval.

Physical examination

The child must be subjected to a routine general examination, but with specific reference to a complete neurological examination. Further special regard should be given to a supplementary neurological examination in children with developmental clumsiness. To the uninitiated the very long list of items which should always be checked in this type of assessment might appear formidable, but the experienced operator would certainly not take more than 15 to 20 minutes to complete this aspect of the assessment.

The general demeanour of the child including behaviour, attitude, attentiveness and general rapport should be noted.

Speech

The assessment of speech function, especially content of speech, in the school-age child is of fundamental importance in the judgement of intellectual function. A false impression may be gained from the child who is unduly shy. The general formulation of speech or phasis should not be disturbed in a child with developmental apraxia unless there is an associated aphasic component to his cortical dysfunctions. There is more usually a defect of articulation and if this is present an attempt should be made to differentiate an apraxia of articulation from a speech defect resulting from an apraxia of the articulatory muscles.

Cerebral dominance

A determination of handedness may be elusive in the ambidextrous child who has not yet learned to write. Some idea of manual dominance might be forthcoming from asking the child to perform a number of tasks such as undoing a safety pin, throwing a ball, or combing the hair. A child will also tend to hop on the dominant foot and to kick a ball with that limb. Cerebral dominance including mixed dominance should be decided by observation of handedness and footedness. Eyedness is a less reliable index of cerebral dominance because the vision of each eye is subserved by both cerebral hemispheres and eye dominance also may be conditioned by refractive error or incipient squint.

Cranial nerves

The most important of cranial nerve functions with regard to educational and general ability in children relates both to visual and hearing acuity. In school medical examination programmes, vision and hearing are recognised as being all important in the general screening of children, but unhappily they are often the least tested of all neurological functions in the consulting room. Because of the important implications of squint in children with clumsiness or disturbance of motor ability due to poor eye–hand co-ordination the clinician should be well versed in a screening assessment of squint. The simple 'cover' test with observation of primary and secondary deviation of the eyes should be carried out in every case.

Motor system

The competence with which the neurological examination is executed is of prime importance in the assessment of tone, power and co-ordination. In this context co-ordination refers to the routine tests carried out in all conventional neurological examinations including the 'finger-nose' test, fine finger movement, 'heel-knee-shin' test and rapid alternating movements (to search for dysdiadochokinesia in the upper and lower limbs). Deep tendon reflex asymmetry or abnormal Babinski responses are amongst the most useful of physical signs as they are characteristic of organic central nervous system dysfunction.

Observations should always be made on the posture of the limbs and the presence of tremor or other abnormal movements. Choreiform movements may indeed be the only observed neurological sign in the assessment of developmental clumsiness.

Sensation

It is often not appreciated how important the assessment of two-point discrimination, joint position sense and stereognosis might be in the assessment of clumsiness in children. Sometimes impairment of these sensory modalities may be severe enough to contribute to observed abnormal movements implicating the presence of pseudoathetosis as a component of sensory ataxia.

Skeletal configuration

The assessment of skull, spinal and limb development is very germane to the issue of the neurological examination. Undue enlargement of the skull might well suggest the presence of a compensated hydrocephalus which should alert the examiner to the possibility of a trivial diplegia. Any departure from the normal shape of the skull might also indicate the presence of an underlying cerebral malformation such as a porencephalic cyst. The presence of pes cavus with or without scoliosis is always of special interest in the neurological examination for it may represent the earliest symptomatology of a progressive heredofamilial spinocerebellar degeneration. Alternatively, these skeletal deformities may occur in association with formes frustes of such conditions as Friedreich's ataxia perhaps with minimal ataxia or lack of motor facility in association with unobtrusively absent ankle jerks. Further important considerations of the axial skeleton include the short neck of the child with the Klippel–Feil deformity which may be associated with underlying spinal cord and brain stem pathology such as syringomyelia, Arnold–Chiari malformation and basilar invagination. Occasionally, Klippel–Feil deformity has been described in association with mirror movements (Ford, 1966) which may in turn be complicated by clumsiness (Crawford, 1960). There should also be careful palpation of the lower lumbar spine for evidence of spina bifida which might occur in conjunction with the so-called 'orthopaedic syndrome' of James and Lassman (1967).

General Examination

No competent clinician would fail to carry out an assessment of the cardiac and respiratory systems and palpation of the abdomen. Chronic disease in any non-neurological system can certainly have a non-specific retarding effect on neurological development.

Supplementary Neurological Examination

Most paediatricians include their own favourite tests in the assessment of a child's motor ability during the course of the examination. The most popular of these include hopping on either leg which is usually possible in pre-school children and walking heel to toe which may not be achieved easily until the age of seven or eight years. Some authorities place importance upon the presence of associated movements (synkinesis) where motor activity in one hand may be mirrored by similar but often less pronounced movement in the other. The implication here is that associated movements have been regarded as an indicator of neurological immaturity. Choreiform movements can be elicited during the time of the routine neurological examination of the motor system. The assessment of finger sense for the presence of finger agnosia is most conveniently tested by the method of Kinsbourne and Warrington (1962). Together with right–left orientation, finger sense may be included in the general assessment of the preservation of the body image. In patients with associated reading disability and problems relating to vision it would be as well to test for oculomotor apraxia (Cogan's syndrome). It is relevant to mention at this point that workers in the field of minimal cerebral dysfunction have sometimes advocated the elicitation of 'soft' neurological signs. A list of these signs is given by Schain (1972), although Ingram (1973) has cautioned against the use of the term.

Reading, Writing and Drawing

Wherever possible the examiner should adopt a set of short standardised tests. Assessment of reading age should not only be the prerogative of the schoolteacher or educational psychologist. The physician should be prepared to carry out this examination in context, and the school medical officer should certainly include this in his routine neurological assessment. It is more difficult to administer or interpret tests of handwriting, but much insight into a child's general abilities can be obtained by examining a sample of handwriting and observing how the child actually manipulates the writing implement. The examiner must also have a fair knowledge of standardised tests of drawing and copying shapes. A sound appreciation of the child's topographical and visuospatial sense may be forthcoming, but should always be checked against similar tests administered by psychologists. Often the child with dressing apraxia will manifest constructional apraxia as evidenced by his inability to copy drawings of simple shapes.

Standardised Tests of Motor Proficiency

There is no doubt that the clinical psychologist is very skilled in assessing motor proficiency and it would be improper for non-psychologically trained personnel to administer psychological tests. On the other hand, the administration of tests of motor proficiency should never be regarded as the exclusive right of the psychological discipline, provided the shortcomings of simpler tests of motor proficiency are appreciated.

The tests described below (Gubbay, 1972) have been developed from the normative data collected in the survey on approximately 1000 schoolchildren described in Chapter 4. These tests are applicable to children aged 8 to 12 years inclusive, and it is these age groups which are most often referred for assessment of developmental clumsiness. However, there is also a definite need for a further development of these tests and standardisation of another set of simple tests for children at the ages of six and seven years. If these tests are carried out reasonably frequently, the experienced examiner can administer the whole battery comprising eight tests in two or three minutes for a well-co-ordinated older child, or in four or five minutes for the average clumsy child. A much longer time would need to be apportioned for the clumsiest children, but this is exceptional.

Tests of Motor Proficiency

(Standardised for children between the ages of 8 and 12 years.)

Test 1—Whistle through pouted lips

The child is required to make a musical note of any pitch and intensity by blowing air through pouted lips.
Score: pass or fail.

Test 2—Skip forward five steps

Three attempts are allowed after demonstration of the test by the examiner (i.e. single hop on left leg, step, single hop on right leg, etc.—without skipping rope).
Score: pass or fail.

Test 3—Roll ball with foot

The child is required to roll a tennis ball under the sole of the preferred foot (with or without footwear) in spiral fashion around 6 matchboxes placed 30 cm apart. The ball is permitted to touch a maximum of 3 matchboxes before disqualification. Three attempts are allowed before failure.
Score: expressed in seconds time or as failure.

Test 4—Throw, clap hands then catch tennis ball

The child is required to clap his hands to a maximum of four times after throwing a tennis ball upwards and catching the ball with both hands. If able to catch the ball after four claps, the child is then required to catch the ball with one (either) hand after four claps. Three attempts are allowed before failure at any point.
Score: expressed in one of the following seven categories:

a. Cannot catch the ball with both hands,
b. Can catch the ball with both hands after 0 claps,
c. Can catch the ball with both hands after 1 clap,
d. Can catch the ball with both hands after 2 claps,
e. Can catch the ball with both hands after 3 claps,
f. Can catch the ball with both hands after 4 claps,
g. Can catch the ball with preferred hand after 4 claps.

Test 5—Tie one shoelace with double bow (single knot)

The examiner's right shoelace with approximately 20-cm lengths protruding from the shoe is offered.
Score: expressed in seconds time or failure if greater than 60 seconds.

Test 6—Thread 10 beads*

The wooden beads are 3 cm in diameter with a bore of 0.8 cm and the terminal 6 cm of the string is stiffened.
Score: expressed in seconds time.

---

* The beads are patented Kiddicraft toys which can be readily purchased.

Test 7—Pierce 20 pinholes

The child is supplied with a stylus (long hatpin) and asked to pierce two successive rows of 1/10th inch × 1/10th inch (2.5 mm × 2.5 mm) squares on graph paper.
Score: expressed in seconds time.

Test 8—Posting box*

The child is required to fit six different plastic shapes in appropriate slots.
Score: expressed in seconds time or failure if greater than 60 seconds.

Method of Scoring

The 5th, 10th, 50th, 90th and 95th percentile values for ages 8, 9, 10, 11 and 12 years are given in Tables 5.1 to 5.5. Scoring may be simplified as follows:
A child may be regarded as below the 5th percentile for his age in motor proficiency if he has three or more scores below the 10th percentile for his age. These 10th percentile values are given in Table 5.6.

Table 5.1. 8-year-olds—screening tests percentiles

Test	5th	10th	50th	90th	95th
1. Whistle	Fail	Fail	Pass	Pass	Pass
2. 5 skips	Fail	Pass	Pass	Pass	Pass
3. Roll ball (seconds)	29	26	19	13	12
4. Catch ball (no. of claps)	1	2	3	4	4
5. Shoelace (seconds)	Fail	Fail	12	8	7
6. 10 beads (seconds)	47	44	34	27	27
7. 20 holes (seconds)	43	39	25	18	17
8. Posting box (seconds)	46	25	14	10	10

Test 5.2. 9-year-olds—screening tests percentiles

Test	5th	10th	50th	90th	95th
1. Whistle	Fail	Fail	Pass	Pass	Pass
2. 5 skips	Fail	Pass	Pass	Pass	Pass
3. Roll ball (seconds)	28	23	16	11	10
4. Catch ball (no. of claps)	2	2	3	4D[a]	4D[a]
5. Shoelace (seconds)	Fail	18	9	7	6
6. 10 beads (seconds)	43	41	32	26	25
7. 20 holes (seconds)	37	31	22	16	14
8. Posting box (seconds)	31	21	13	10	9

[a] D = Dominant hand.

---

* The posting box is a patented Kiddicraft toy which can be readily purchased.

Table 5.3. 10-year-olds—screening tests percentiles

Test	5th	10th	50th	90th	95th
1. Whistle	Fail	Fail	Pass	Pass	Pass
2. 5 skips	Fail	Pass	Pass	Pass	Pass
3. Roll ball (seconds)	28	22	14	10	10
4. Catch ball (no. of claps)	2	3	4	4D	4D
5. Shoelace (seconds)	18	14	9	6	6
6. 10 beads (seconds)	39	37	29	25	23
7. 20 holes (seconds)	31	29	21	14	13
8. Posting box (seconds)	21	18	12	9	9

Table 5.4. 11-year-olds—screening tests percentiles

Test	5th	10th	50th	90th	95th
1. Whistle	Fail	Fail	Pass	Pass	Pass
2. 5 skips	Fail	Pass	Pass	Pass	Pass
3. Roll ball (seconds)	20	18	12	10	9
4. Catch ball (no. of claps)	2	3	4	4D	4D
5. Shoelace (seconds)	16	13	9	6	6
6. 10 beads (seconds)	39	37	28	24	23
7. 20 holes (seconds)	29	26	18	13	12
8. Posting box (seconds)	21	18	11	9	8

Table 5.5. 12-year-olds—screening tests percentiles

Test	5th	10th	50th	90th	95th
1. Whistle	Fail	Pass	Pass	Pass	Pass
2. 5 skips	Pass	Pass	Pass	Pass	Pass
3. Roll ball (seconds)	18	17	12	9	8
4. Catch ball (no. of claps)	3	3	4D	4D	4D
5. Shoelace (seconds)	13	11	8	6	5
6. 10 beads (seconds)	34	32	27	23	22
7. 20 holes (seconds)	28	25	17	13	11
8. Posting box (seconds)	26	18	11	8	8

Table 5.6. 10th percentile values

Test	8	9	10	11	12
			Age (years)		
1. Whistle	Fail	Fail	Fail	Fail	Pass
2. 5 skips	Pass	Pass	Pass	Pass	Pass
3. Roll ball (seconds)	26	23	22	18	17
4. Clap and catch ball (no. of claps)	2	2	3	3	3
5. Tie shoelace (seconds)	Fail	18	14	13	11
6. Thread 10 beads (seconds)	44	41	37	37	32
7. Pierce 20 holes (seconds)	39	31	29	26	25
8. Posting box (seconds)	25	21	18	18	18

Reproduced with the kind permission of the editor of *Proceedings of the Australian Association of Neurologists*.

Referrals for Further Assessment

Any suspicion of a progressive neurological disorder should be followed up by referral to a neurologist or paediatric neurologist who would need to bear in mind a differential diagnosis as incorporated in Chapter 1. The presence of conventional neurological signs or a past history of significant neurological illness might also merit a full neurological assessment.

Electroencephalogram

The value of this investigation is discussed fully elsewhere in this book. EEG should not be regarded as a routine investigational tool in patients with developmental clumsiness. Often children are referred for the investigation to help reassure the parents, but in the average case, such a reason is not valid because a considerable proportion of even normal children have 'abnormal' electroencephalograms. The very parent that the clinician hopes to reassure with electroencephalography by proving the innocuous nature of a neurodevelopmental dysfunction is the one most likely to be unduly upset by any mention of an insignificant EEG aberration.

Skull X-ray

Sometimes skull radiography can be employed as a useful instrument for further reassurance and is preferable to electroencephalography in this regard. It should not be used as a routine procedure in neurological assessment unless the child is prone to troublesome headaches. Fortunately in the case of developmental clumsiness, a spurious, equivocal or unexpected finding is unusual. It is certainly wiser to reserve this investigation for cases where there is genuine clinical concern about the possibility of a progressive or serious neurological disorder. It should be carried out in all instances of enlargement of the skull circumference to above the 97th percentile, as the x-ray may yield collateral evidence to adduce the presence of a compensated or arrested hydrocephalus. Skull x-rays also should be considered when the differential diagnosis includes such outside possibilities as raised intracranial pressure, space-occupying lesions, or neurological conditions which may induce intracranial calcification or increased vascularity.

Psychological Tests

In the entire field of assessment in minimal cerebral dysfunction, learning disabilities and in particular developmental clumsiness, the clinical psychologist may play a dominant role. Indeed in this situation the physician might assume a supportive function to the educational psychologist or educationist who may need a medical appraisal before proceeding with an educational programme. The Wechsler Intelligence Scale for Children has been the single most useful psychological test in the assessment of clumsy children. In general, the performance IQ score will turn out to be significantly lower than the verbal IQ. When the developmental apraxia also affects speech function or there is an associated developmental dysarthria, the verbal IQ score may actually be lower than the performance score. The clinical psychologist generally excels in providing valuable information regarding the extent and causation of the child's behaviour. A recognition of frank visuospatial problems may explain secondary behaviour disorders in a child who is unduly stressed by this disability. Alternatively, a psychologist will often throw further light upon a background of social or psychological turmoil which may have a secondary retarding effect on a child's specific learning ability in one or other category.

SUMMARY

A full assessment of the clumsy child requires a complete neurological appraisal. In most instances it would be ideal for this type of assessment to be made by school medical officers, as part of the medical service offered to schoolchildren. After obtaining a full history relating to the specific deficiencies of the child, special inquiry should be made into the developmental, past and psychiatric histories. Other routine historical factors concerned in the medical assessment of children detailed above should not be overlooked. A competent neurological examination need not necessarily be carried out by a neurologist and indeed the average adult neurologist may be less informed about the administration and significance of useful supplementary neurological tests than the paediatrician, or a specially trained school medical officer. The physician should also include the assessment of Reading Age as part of his own responsibility. His testing armamentarium should include a battery of simple standardised tests of motor proficiency. Such a test battery together with normative data is fully described and offered for use here.

Supporting information should be forthcoming from clinical psychologists. Investigational tools include the electroencephalogram and skull x-ray in selected cases.

The eight tests for motor proficiency suggested in this section may be used for the assessment of individual children but their usefulness can also be extended to the screening of large numbers of children for the presence of defective motor skills.

Accuracy and attention to detail in the assessment of the clumsy child is an important prerequisite to effective management.

CHAPTER SIX

Management

It is not possible for any one individual to assume total responsibility for the clumsy child. Quite apart from the considerations of diagnosis and assessment, the task of helping the child with his or her specific problem usually requires the co-ordinated effort of several individuals, each from varying professional disciplines. The interdisciplinary approach has been stressed by many workers in the field of minimal cerebral dysfunction, and specific learning disability. However, there can never be a clearly stated policy as to which particular discipline should be ultimately responsible for the co-ordination of effort in any one particular case. Clearly the medical practitioner cannot be expected to determine matters of educational policy. The educational psychologist, schoolteacher or therapist in varying instances may be able to assume individual dominant roles in management. Whilst the interdependence between the various professional groups may be a healthy attitude, this may occur at the expense of a clear orientation for the relatively unsophisticated parent.

The medical advisor should assume the dominant co-ordinating role when the greatest anxiety is centred upon aetiological or behavioural considerations. We all tend to look to the educationist for overall guidance when the predominant feature happens to be failure at school. However, the educationist does not have at his disposal the facility to refer the child for specific therapy, e.g. speech therapy, psychotherapy, etc. Although the general medical practitioner should not be discouraged from assuming a co-ordinating role, in most instances he cannot be expected to cope with the niceties of interdisciplinary assessment and management. Until a more satisfactory solution can be reached, the neurologist or paediatrician is likely to be the individual to whom parents will ultimately turn for advice. Ideally, the type of person required for this job would be a medically qualified individual, capable of carrying out a competent neurological assessment with a clear appreciation of neurodevelopmental dysfunctions and a good working knowledge of educational principles. We can reasonably expect that this type of physician will emerge from our present school medical services. To this end it should be possible to institute in-service courses for current school medical officers who could then be expected to concentrate more on individual assessments of children than on screening procedures. He would also be in an ideal situation to co-ordinate the assessments by the neurologist, paediatrician, orthopaedic surgeon, ophthalmologist, ear nose and throat specialist, therapist and educational psychologist and to utilise this information to guide the individual schoolteacher or headmaster towards some of the educational principles which might be appropriate in any one particular child's case.

Conservatism has a definite part to play in the treatment of children with specific clumsiness, but it should not be confused with therapeutic nihilism. In many cases an expectant approach by parents, teachers and doctors might be rewarded in time by spontaneous improvement. It is often very difficult to predict which child has maturational lag and eventually will improve spontaneously as opposed to the child requiring specific educational therapy. A conservative approach should be adopted wherever the doubt exists, but when the environmental requirements are so competitive it may be discreet if not expedient to reduce the pressures on a child and institute some modifications in management.

The preventative aspects of treatment are no less important in the field of developmental clumsiness than in any other therapeutic situation. All writers on the subject of the management of the clumsy child or allied disturbances emphasise the importance of early diagnosis, not only for the sake of an early institution of therapeutic measures, but also to avoid unpleasant repercussions on the misunderstood child.

Whilst early diagnosis has a preventative aspect, ultimate prevention must be applied mainly through epidemiological principles. Optimal care during the perinatal period, adequate nutrition during infancy and childhood, and a move towards the enrichment of backgrounds of culturally deprived children are three separate issues which require further discussion. Firstly, the improvement of perinatal care might on the one hand prevent some children from minor degrees of anoxic birth injury, or spare children from a severe to a milder category of cerebral dysfunction, but on the other hand will allow the survival of children who might otherwise have had potentially fatal conditions. As long as there are a significant number of children with anoxic birth injury, an improvement in the management of pregnancy, delivery and neonatal period will not reduce the total number of children with minimal cerebral dysfunction, but it should reduce their proportion compared with normal children. Secondly, undernutrition and other forms of malnutrition are not always the result of poor economic circumstances. An adequate understanding of simple principles with regard to nutrition is lacking even in countries with advanced living standards. The third preventative consideration, namely in the field of enrichment programmes for the culturally deprived, is a contentious issue. Regimentation of children into preschool programmes may have a certain benefit on the deprived minority with a potentially deleterious effect on the development of individuality in the undeprived majority. These broad social issues are ultimately the responsibility of epidemiological advisors to governments. The possible role of genetic counselling in families of children with developmental anomalies should not be overlooked. Children with emotional or physical handicaps also must be included amongst those to whom a preventative approach is necessary.

Although the role of the paediatrician and neurologist may be mainly in the fields of assessment and diagnosis with regard to the clumsy child, they have the very special responsibility of communicating the diagnosis and its implications to both the parent and the child. Until a special rationalisation of management by a specific agency such as a school medical service is forthcoming the specialist physician should also be responsible for further communication with a child's schoolteacher, headmaster, educational guidance officer, and paramedical therapists. He may well have to utilise the potential reassurance of special investigational studies such as the skull x-ray and electroencephalogram and the latter may be of importance with respect to drug therapy. Part of his responsibility applies to advice regarding the parental care of the child in the home environment and he may have to give psychological support to both parent and child. He may be in a position to advise regarding sporting activities at school and the classroom situation when it applies to physical tasks, such as handwriting, drawing, modelling, sewing and other manual arts and crafts. The remedial teacher will often be grateful for meaningful contact with the medical profession whose opinion in turn may well be sought with regard to the institution of specific therapies and remedial motor programmes. The physician must be responsible for the integration of paramedical personnel in deploying the services of speech therapist, occupational therapist and physiotherapist. His ultimate responsibility may lie within the field of vocational guidance when his advice will take prognosis into account.

THE MEDICAL SPECIALIST

The mode of presentation to the paediatrician or the neurologist will usually be through referral from another medical practitioner. The instigation of such referral will nearly always be by an anxious parent who may have been advised accordingly by the schoolteacher, remedial teacher, or school medical officer to obtain neurological assessment and advice.

The responsibility of the specialist carrying out the neurological assessment lies primarily in the field of diagnosis. After considering the history of clumsiness and performing a full routine neurological examination, the informed clinician will also carry out a supplementary neurological examination during the course of the physical assessment. He may search for 'soft signs' even though their significance might be dubious. In any case, he should make an assessment of hand and foot dominance and determine whether crossed cerebral dominance is present. When testing for right—left orientation and finger sense it should be realised that most children do not develop these facilities until sometime after the age of seven years. It is also conventional to test the child's ability to hop on either leg, to jump and to copy finger postures. It is mandatory for the physician to test the child's handwriting to dictation and spatial sense in copying drawings such as a clock-face. The physician now has access to a series of standardised tests of motor proficiency which can be rapidly executed and which has been devised specially for the medical practitioner in this context (see Chapter 5).

Psychometric evaluation of the child should probably always be sought. The educational psychologist will usually choose a combination of test batteries before making a final formulation, but the less experienced psychologist if seeking guidance might well be advised to administer the WISC. Much reassurance can be gained when it is known that the deficiency in motor skills does not reflect an overall subnormal intellect.

By this time the physician, taking the social history into consideration, will be in a position to know whether there has been any emotional or cultural deprivation contributing to the overall problem of clumsiness. He should be able to judge whether any emotional disorder could have been an important contributory agent in the child's presentation. In these circumstances it is very much the physician's responsibility to attempt some modification of the social and cultural environment. If this is beyond his own resources, he should enlist the aid of the social worker. In some cases he should ensure further referral to a psychiatrist working in the field and who has at his disposal specific agencies for dealing with sociocultural problems.

INTERVIEWING THE CHILD

After obtaining the child's confidence, possibly at a subsequent consultation, it is desirable that the physician communicates directly with a diagnostic formulation. These few moments spent in counselling the child may be far more valuable than leaving the parent or schoolteacher to explain a diagnosis secondhand. Naturally, the orientation of this particular aspect of the interview should be one towards reassurance explaining that the physical problem exists through no personal fault of the child and that it is amenable to treatment. It has been advocated that even the demonstration of a minimal sign to the parent or child might have a salutary effect. The aim should also be to dispel from the child's mind any fears that may have developed as the result of extensive medical and psychological assessments. Due cognisance must be given to the child's individuality. He should not be regarded as a mere passive test object which happens to be the substrate of an intellectual exercise by the physician as a service rendered to parents. Sometimes the overprotective parent may wish to exclude the child from much of the interview. Wherever possible this attitude should be actively discouraged by gently expounding upon the dangers of puerile misapprehensions. In the test situations, the unfortunate subject often exposes the entire depth of his or her disabilities to the point of embarrassment which might not be immediately apparent. A few words of encouragement may do much to obviate the possibility of loss of self-esteem.

INTERVIEWING THE PARENT

More than in other fields of paediatric assessment, it is not really possible to make a proper evaluation of a child's disabilities without the attendance of a parent. The child's environmental influences come readily into focus after the initial interview. It is not surprising that most of the children referred to clinicians for clumsiness and related disorders are offspring of relatively high achievers in the community. Not only do these parents tend to have higher aspirations for their children, but the relative disabilities of these children are highlighted against a background of greater adeptness and competence in friends and siblings. Psychological, social and cultural problems directly due to parental influence may not be treatable by the clinician, but frank discussion of these issues may help the parent to formulate a resourceful plan of action.

The care of the general health of the child is an obvious factor of management, and attention to the correction of chronic illnesses may do much to improve attention span and concentration. There should be an avoidance of unnecessary fatigue, for example from late nights, long excursions to the city, and prolonged periods of inactivity in strained circumstances predisposing to a subsequent emotional release of frustration. Sometimes the interaction between the child and parent may result in undue strain on the parent. This is more likely to occur in perfectionistic parents with obsessional traits who would become utterly frustrated by the lack of responsiveness of their children to repeated attempts at physical training at home. It may not be sufficient to discourage actively this type of parent from adding insult to injury. Sometimes benefit can accrue from reducing the strain on these parents by encouraging baby-sitting or even arranging for trained babysitters who are able to cope with any special complicating problems such as hyperactivity.

One of the more important factors of home management is to reduce the pressures on the child to conform to the norms of motor function such as sporting skills, drawing and especially handwriting. Wherever possible the child with specific problems should be given a separate room with tranquil surroundings. There could be danger of overstimulation from numerous toys requiring continual maintenance by indexterous fingers such as electric trains. Firm and consistent maintenance of discipline should be balanced against allowing the child to be alone either indoors or outdoors where he can develop his own individuality.

The parent should be encouraged to communicate his or her anxieties regarding the child to the headmaster and the class schoolteacher. The demanding parent often becomes unduly frustrated by insisting upon special facilities which cannot be forthcoming without overburdening the school's resources.

ELECTROENCEPHALOGRAPHY

Electroencephalography is a much abused investigation in the field of minimal cerebral dysfunction, specific learning disability and in developmental clumsiness in particular. It is unfortunate that the clinician will often yield to pressures to carry out this apparently harmless investigation by the parent who sometimes has been advised to this end by paramedical personnel. They may feel that the investigation casts a wider net which might occasionally bring unsuspected abnormalities to light. The clinician recognising the procedure as innocuous and anticipating a normal result might unwittingly incite more parental anxiety by giving unconvincing reassurances about 'minor abnormalities'. The more astute physician, particularly one with electroencephalographic experience, will often warn the parent of the vagaries of EEG reporting and jargon. He should anticipate all contingencies by clearly stating at the outset that an abnormality would have to be significant before taking it into consideration. EEG changes which may be regarded as significant include unequivocal epileptiform phenomena, persistent rhythm asymmetries and pronounced focal changes or progressive abnormalities. Thus the EEG is a useful adjunct in progressive or focal disease. An important aspect of electroencephalography is to assist in the management of drug therapy.

DRUG THERAPY

Although drug treatment does not directly influence physical co-ordination of children with developmental clumsiness, drugs will sometimes favourably influence overall performance through their beneficial effects on hyperactivity, anxiety, depression and seizure disorders. Children with developmental clumsiness have a higher incidence of paroxysmal and epileptiform EEG changes than the population at large. Where the clinical history suggests minor seizures or seizure equivalents the necessity for anticonvulsant medication is indisputable. Where there is no such history, but the EEG exhibits convincing evidence of epileptiform dysrhythmia, the clinician should always be tempted to make a trial of anticonvulsants. In cases of juvenile migraine, where there is associated EEG dysrhythmia (dysrhythmic headache) or non-specific behaviour disorders associated with epileptiform activity, anticonvulsant medication has always been advocated. Occasionally anticonvulsants can produce a remarkable improvement in apparent integrative cerebral function, but this is exceptional. In general, barbiturate drugs such as phenobarbitone should be assiduously avoided even in children with epilepsy as there is a great tendency for them to aggravate problems of hyperactivity and generally difficult behaviour (Bradley, 1937; Ingram, 1956; Conners and Eisenberg, 1963; Baldwin and Kenny, 1966; Eisenberg, 1966; Millichap and Boldrey, 1967; Millichap and Fowler, 1967; Millichap et al, 1968).

In subjects with overt epilepsy it is an accepted principle of treatment to titrate the drug dosage against the clinical response having due regard for unpleasant side effects. Where there is no such clear guideline to the level of dosage in children with minimal cerebral dysfunction, it is worth checking the plasma drug levels. Gas chromatographic methods have facilitated drug level estimations of diphenylhydantoin (Dilantin, Epanutin) and carbamazepine (Tegretol). In cases where there are prominent EEG abnormalities, the investigation may be a useful method of monitoring drug dosage.

In children with hyperactivity, the apparently paradoxical sedative action of some of the central nervous system stimulant drugs may have a beneficial effect. Other psychotropic medications including tranquilliser drugs may be more useful in many instances. Central nervous system stimulants have been recommended as the agents of choice by Millichap (1973) in children with minimal brain dysfunction. The two cerebral stimulants presently in usage, namely dexamphetamine (Dexedrine) and methylphenidate (Ritalin), are superior to other drugs in the control of hyperactivity, impulsivity and aggression and improvement of attention span, co-ordination and visual and auditory perception. Although these drugs are less likely to produce drowsiness than other psychotropic agents they may result in anorexia and troublesome weight loss. Occasionally, although behaviour may be more tractable as in the classroom, there may be unacceptable personality changes. Schain (1972) has recommended that methylphenidate be given in an initial dose of 5 to 10 mg or dexamphetamine 2.5 to 5 mg. Therapeutic effects may not occur until there has been a gradual increase of dosage of methylpenidate up to 80 mg per day or dexamphetamine to 40 mg per day. These drugs should usually be given in divided doses morning and noon, taking care to administer them after meals unless the child is overweight. It has been assumed that amphetamines and other drugs such as methylphenidate and tricyclic antidepressants facilitate the synaptic effects of brain catecholamines (Snyder and Meyerhoff, 1973). The alerting effect of these drugs may be mediated by the influence of the brainstem reticular formation on cerebral arousal mechanisms. The mutual interdependence of alertness and muscle co-ordination have specific application to the problem of developmental clumsiness. Deanol (Deaner), another central nervous stimulant, has not been shown to be of value in the treatment of hyperactive behaviour and learning disabilities despite the low incidence of side effects (Millichap, 1973). A full discussion on the usefulness of alternative drugs such as chlordiazepoxide (Librium), thioridazine (Melleril, Mellaril), chlorpromazine (Largactil, Thorazine), reserpine (Serpasil) and imipramine (Tofranil) is also discussed by Millichap (1973). Occasionally antidepressant drugs may be needed when the child has developed a depressed state of mind.

When drugs are instituted in the treatment of children with developmental clumsiness and associated behavioural anomalies, there must be adequate liaison with the child's schoolteachers and therapists. In many cases an enthusiastic remedial teacher making progress with a particular child might well ask for medication to be deferred. An adequate feedback regarding the effects of the drug on fidgetiness in the classroom, general co-ordination, behaviour and overall school performance is a fundamental requirement for the responsible clinician. Wherever possible one should try and obtain the child's own opinion of taking medication, if only to dispel undue anxiety or undesirable misapprehensions regarding drug taking. Solomons (1973) warns against the frequently inaccurate information given by parents and teachers as well as the possible placebo effects on a child. There may be undue overreaction by a schoolteacher who feels that there should be an alteration of the drug regimen. Other hazards of drug administration are discussed and these include cost, parent reliability, availability of addictive drugs to delinquent siblings, placebo effects, unknown effects of long-term medication, misdiagnosis and injudicious use of medication. Wherever possible clinicians should allow some time for the monitoring of drug dosage by telephone to obviate the need for multiple visits.

INTERDEPARTMENTAL COMMUNICATION

With parental consent the physician has a particular responsibility to communicate wherever possible, especially with educational authorities at all levels. Direct contact is necessary as communication through the medium of a parent may not only be unreliable, but might foster unnecessary resentment on both sides. A simple telephone call to the headmaster or a short note to the class teacher or school medical officer are likely to result in much greater co-operation with a significant easing of the burden of responsibility on the parent. The overprotectiveness of some teachers and a resentment of interference by others can sometimes be prevented by a co-operative approach. The class teacher, whilst respecting the professional confidence between parent and doctor, may feel unduly isolated. Due cognisance should be given to the fact that the schoolteacher spends infinitely more time thinking about the child's problems than the clinician and is often more perturbed about genuine difficulties with a child than his or her parents.

EDUCATIONAL CONSIDERATIONS

General Observations

At the present time it is still relatively uncommon for children with an isolated developmental apraxia to present as a specific educational problem. Clumsiness in itself is of secondary importance to the educational therapist who is primarily concerned with more fundamental defects of learning ability as it applies specifically to reading, writing, spelling and mathematics. The remedial teacher soon becomes aware that a large number of children with learning problems have an associated clumsiness. He or she is unlikely to be presented with a child with good reading or mathematical ability, but who is maladroit at physical tasks unless the latter greatly interferes with writing ability. Thus developmental clumsiness in isolation is somewhat lower on the list of priorities with regard to remediation because it interferes with a child's formal education much less than communication skills. Educational authorities therefore are likely to consider clumsiness as part of a wider problem requiring remedial teaching. In any case, whether the clumsiness of developmental apraxia presents as a specific feature or whether it is part of the total symptom complex of minimal cerebral dysfunction (with or without specific learning disability), the same principles of remediation must apply. Remedial educational methods for specific learning disabilities in general are outside the scope of this book.

One of the more important principles pertaining to specific educational therapy in these children is not so much *what* is being done for the child, but more that *something* is being done. Bringing the child into focus by the recognition of his problem immediately reduces the pressures to conform. The major ingredient of a successful programme is "a learning environment that provides a measure of protection for the child until such time as a higher level of central nervous system maturity and integration can be achieved, most probably by the natural course of time" (Clements and Peters, 1973). "When no-progress plateaus are reached, the teacher, as well as others, must operate with the understanding that the plateaus are not her fault, but that she should temporarily abandon the big push for presently unattainable skills". These principles apply whether the child remains in a regular classroom wherein modifications are made in the curriculum and management or whether the child attends special classrooms or special schools.

Initially the choice of school may be fundamental as much depends upon the facilities at the particular school whether it be government or privately run. Ideally, classes should be reasonably small if the child is to be integrated into a normal classroom. In special classrooms there should probably not be more than 10 or 15 pupils and the teacher in attendance should be trained in special education methods. These teachers should be specially selected because of the importance of the personality, temperament and skill of the individual. We may eventually be able to reach the ideal situation where the educational programme is planned by an educational therapist who might apply prescriptive or individualised treatment. Short teaching sessions may be necessary for the short attention spans and the teacher might need to teach to the child's strengths rather than to his weaknesses. It would be necessary to adopt an understanding attitude that the child's errors are unintentional and are unavoidable and the child should be given concessions for slow, untidy handwriting. Simple physical tasks entrusted to the child such as erasing the blackboard may improve his self-esteem and confidence. After the age of 11 or 12 years, it may be reasonable to teach the child to type in order to circumvent some of the problems which may come with handwriting. Detailed recommendations for classroom procedures are given by Rogan and Lukens (1969).

An attractively pragmatic approach to teaching methods for children with special problems is expounded by Cohen (1973). Diagnostic and aetiological labels are apparently of no real practical importance to the educator because "All people, learning disabled or not, are subject to certain universal laws of learning". He has outlined a number of interacting principles pertaining to the laws of learning. Thus, feedback should be paced, immediate and positive. This feedback should reinforce the appropriate stimulus condition in short, learning modules. When these principles are not applied to a specific response, one cannot expect learning to occur.

The retarding effect of deprivation on motor development has been described by Dennis (1941) who showed that although deprivation delayed development, subsequent practice rapidly raised the level of the child's achievements up to but not beyond his potential. Brenner et al (1967) have recognised the urgent need for research into the degree to which visuomotor disability (which may lead to clumsiness) may be overcome or compensated by appropriate remedial training. Kass, Hall and Simches (1969) have looked into the question of legislative assistance in the management of the problem of minimal cerebral dysfunction. Other authors have alluded to the various principles involved in the educational and general management of the clumsy child within the context of minimal cerebral dysfunction (Ounsted, 1955; Bakwin and Bakwin, 1960; Wigglesworth, 1963; Cohn, 1964; Bakwin, 1968a;

Bateman and Schiefelbusch, 1969; Gallagher et al, 1969; Haring, Reid and Beaber, 1969; Masland, 1969a).

The Classroom Situation

Special qualities are a fundamental requirement of the individual teacher of children with specific problems. It is asserted here that the chance of worthwhile improvement is greatly diminished when there is no sense of dedication or enthusiasm. No amount of intellectualisation or theorising can be a substitute for the sympathetic one to one relationship between teacher and pupil. In some instances of deprivation of motor experience, the child may benefit by mere exposure to a variety of motor activities. This type of child with normal potential should improve rapidly by supplementing his impoverished home background with extra school facilities such as bicycle riding, game puzzles and drawing materials. Some teachers will resort to finding out the point where there has been a breakdown in the child's motor skills. When the area of breakdown has been identified, she is then in the position to apply a hierarchy of motor tasks from more gross to finer movements.

Although the beneficial practice effect of constant repetition at a task poorly performed might be a fundamental learning principle it may be wiser to employ parallel exercises. For instance, a child with particularly untidy handwriting should be encouraged to write with chalk on the blackboard or to use scissors. When one type of programme appears to be unsuccessful the teacher should have no hesitation in switching to an alternative programme at least for a time. A prime consideration should always be a reduction of tensions on the child as this will nearly always be rewarded by improved motor performance.

An improvement of spatial awareness and left—right orientation may be of particular advantage. The children should not only be encouraged to exercise in their physical training periods, but also to develop a sense of topographical orientation and of body awareness.

The pioneering efforts of Albitreccia (1958, 1959) are still held in high regard from the practical point of view in the treatment of disorders of the body image. She was able to recognise disturbances of body image in children suffering from motor disorders. A number of therapeutic exercises had been advocated. These included the exploration of the body by touching, naming and moving its component parts with the aid of pictures and diagrams, and the construction of a face from its separate elements. The awareness of the body in space was facilitated by simulating postures adopted by a manikin and by modelling clay images. Other types of constructive activity advocated were cutting out from cardboard and carrying out exercises requiring ideational praxis. The formulation of letters and rhythm therapy were also described together with the use of graded exercises for which a special apparatus was required. Further techniques in this regard have been described by McAninch (1966).

The applications of operant conditioning to the development of motor skill in children has been discussed by Connolly (1968). The therapist imposes a stimulus on the child in an attempt to bring about a response under stimulus control. It is necessary for this type of system to possess three factors including: (1) reward; (2) information regarding performance (feedback); and (3) motivation. Reinforcement by sounds and tape-recorded messages are helpful, but kinaesthetic feedback although important is difficult to devise mechanically. In general there needs to be a systematised programme of rhythmic and sensory activity.

The child with agnosia and apraxia demands patient individual attention (Ellis, 1967). He may need to be taught how to hold a knife and fork or cup, how to manipulate doorknobs or doorhandles and how to dress and undress himself. At an early stage the teaching of these hand skills may be deemed to be within the province of an occupational therapist. Other factors that might need special instruction include walking up and down stairs and ball throwing and catching. There is a need for constant repetition of these motor activities which call for a great deal of patience on the part of the child and of those who are trying to help him. Graded developmental exercises have been advocated by Hatton (1966). Thus, the child with reading and writing problems may be hampered by poorly developed gross motor skills and such a child should be placed on a schedule which includes passive and/or active exercises involving balancing, ball rolling, creeping, throwing balls or tossing rings. A useful plan of action is also given for some therapy by parents.

The Doman–Delacato treatment of neurologically handicapped children has received much unfavourable publicity (*Developmental Medicine and Child Neurology,* 1968). The therapy is said to be based on questionable oversimplified concepts of hemispheric dominance and the relation of individual sequential development to phylogenesis. The methods have been very seriously challenged as the validity of the technique has been unsubstantiated (Delacato, 1963; Freeman, 1967; Robbins, 1967).

A critical evaluation of remedial programmes is still forthcoming (Skatvedt, 1963; Hawke, 1971). An excellent detailed review on management in minimal brain dysfunction is given by Miller (1969) and valid points in this regard have also been made by Anderson and Plymate (1962), Paine (1968), Reuben and Bakwin (1968) and Dare and Gordon (1970).

The Sporting Field

Alas, nothing is more humiliating to the apraxic child than his desultory efforts on the sporting field or in the gymnasium. He may become so discouraged by his repeated failure, especially if he becomes an object of hilarity, that his sportsmaster may be content to allow him to recline on the sidelines. Truancy by these children on sportsday is likely to occur or the child may rationalise his problems by purporting to be ill at these times. The problem can sometimes be solved in larger schools where there may be a greater variety of sports from which to choose. These children are probably best encouraged to take up rugby rather than soccer in winter and swimming and athletics rather than tennis or cricket in summer. Although similar principles should apply in the case of girls, in general they are not subjected to the same sociocultural pressures to achieve any degree of excellence at sport. Because it is so important for these clumsy children to be included in team games wherever possible, the physical education teacher should be prepared to place them in a position of lesser responsibility on the field and to lend a watchful and protective eye to obviate the danger of injury. Just as the remedial teacher is expected to spend a little extra time and effort with certain children, sometimes out of normal school hours, so should there be provision for remedial physical education. The popularity of boys adept at sport with their schoolmasters is a well-recognised phenomenon, but an increased exposure of the apraxic child to his physical education instructor is likely to facilitate a more beneficial relationship with the child, restoring some of his self-esteem.

Physical Education

Educationists have adopted a pragmatic approach towards compensatory education or remediation in children with motor impairment. In considering what constitutes a skill it is possible to analyse the component factors. It may be feasible to determine the deficient components of a particular skill which is lacking in a child and it is reasonable to assume that exercises could be devised which would develop a specific skill.

At present it would appear to be an impossible task to determine the relative efficacies of differing remedial exercises. Gross variables make objective assessment extremely difficult; the most important variable being the quality of the teacher. Indeed the teacher may be more important than the actual methodology. Masland (1969) neatly explains the fallacy of specific treatments producing improvements in uncontrolled studies, i.e. when controls were instituted it seemed evident that special attention rather than exercise improved IQ scores in a group of mentally retarded boys. "Despite the many contributions that perceptual-motor programmes make, we cannot overlook the possibility that the major contributions may be psychological and emotional" (Stein, 1971).

Morris and Whiting (1971) provide a description of compensatory education which embodies the approaches of both Frostig (1971) and Kephart (1971). At present physical educationists are concerned largely with the development of general physical and sporting ability. There now would appear to be a move towards specialisation in the treatment of neurologically handicapped children including those with specific learning problems (Fait, 1972).

SPECIFIC THERAPIES

Speech Therapy

Children with developmental apraxia and agnosia have a high incidence of developmental speech disorders. Developmental dysarthria may manifest either as a result of a true apraxia for speech which occurs at a higher level of effector organisation than dysarthria due to apraxia of the muscles of articulation. The speech therapist would be expected to apply the usual principles of treatment to these children with the full recognition of parallel problems of motor dysfunction resulting in clumsiness.

Physiotherapy

The physiotherapist's role usually falls short of treatment of children with developmental apraxia and agnosia. However apraxic difficulties are common in children with congenital encephalopathies ('cerebral palsy'). In many instances the therapist is reliant upon a eupraxic state for the institution of specific exercises. The experienced therapist usually has worked out a programme which facilitates the child's rehabilitation taking into account the super-added apraxic difficulties attributable to intellectual inferiority. The prevention of contractures and facilitation of strength are important principles in the treatment of children with spasticity and abnormal movements, but the physiotherapist may make an even greater contribution with exercises designed to improve appreciation of the body image. In this particular field, physiotherapist, occupational therapist and schoolteacher will overlap in their responsibilities and it may be other considerations which will usually dictate whom the dominant therapist should be.

Orthoptics

The orthoptist may encounter undue difficulty in the apraxic child who is likely to have a higher incidence of squint than normal children. The rare association of congenital oculomotor apraxia with developmental apraxia may not be amenable to orthoptic treatment particularly in younger age groups. Where the disability is relatively mild, the orthoptist may be in a position to devise eye exercises which facilitate the supranuclear control of eye movement.

Occupational Therapy

The role of the occupational therapist in dealing with children who have apraxic problems in cerebral palsy institutions is established. It is likely to be a contentious issue as to whether the occupational therapist has something to offer over and above the remedial teacher at normal or special schools. Certainly, she would be in a good position to give some assistance to the apraxic child on an outpatient basis at a children's hospital. Where a protracted one to one relationship between the child and therapist is required, the occupational therapist may be able to make a real contribution at a remedial school. A clearer appreciation of the overall clinical problem is likely to be forthcoming from the occupational therapist than the remedial teacher.

There would be less disruption of the classroom situation if the child were to be transferred for a period of half an hour or so for special treatment. Wolfik (1973) has drawn attention to the scope of occupational therapy in the early identification, assessment and treatment of the child with minimal brain dysfunction.

A masterly review of the neurophysiological background to learning disorders is given by Ayres (1972a). The explanations in terms of physiology are logical and attractive. The theories expounded for the application of specific therapies are philosophically convincing. Whilst the neurologist is entitled to be more circumspect about her theories of Sensory Integrative Therapy, she does make a genuine attempt at an empirical evaluation of her methods (Ayres, 1972b). An eclectic approach to therapy should include the various activities advocated by her. Amongst the various exercises which have been suggested to develop praxis are included scooter board activities where the child lies in various postures carrying out certain physical tasks on a small mobile platform. The child may be made to roll up in a rug with head and feet arising at designated places or to squirm through a tube of cotton cloth or nylon net, or to walk along a twisted rope on the ground with one foot on either side. Several other activities are described utilising such equipment as a rocking board, large therapy ball, and quadruped balancing board. The act of soft brushing over the child has been regarded as beneficial. These methods would certainly appear to require further evaluation and the test of time.

Prognosis

Ford (1966), in discussing 'Congenital Maladroitness', stated "... having spent much time and effort in learning a certain activity, such as riding a bicycle, the child may eventually perform normally ... They are usually not handicapped in adult life for they choose a business in which muscular coordination is not important." Improvement with increasing maturity has been referred to by Brain and Walton (1969) and Paine (1968) has felt that clumsiness tends to improve just as co-ordination improves in normal children with increasing age. He assumed that perhaps one meets every day on the street many people who formerly fell into the category of minimal cerebral dysfunction, but who are not much different from everyone else once the demand of education pressures are over. They may be slightly awkward adults, they may be socially ill at ease or less successful than their siblings, but nevertheless must have made some reasonably satisfactory adjustment.

Dare and Gordon (1970) have remarked on the lack of comprehensive long-term follow-up studies on these children, but have observed beyond doubt that improvement in skilled movements can occur in a relatively short space of time even in children of below average intelligence. With Bakwin's (1968a) definition of 'developmental delay', it is implicit that recovery of normal function will become complete as opposed to the implications of the notion of 'developmental abnormality'. Gesell and Amatruda (1947) described distinct improvement to the point of appearing almost normal in these children as they grew older.

Masland (1969a) felt that prognosis was dependent to a certain extent upon management and maintained that with special instruction, appropriate to the specific characteristics of the individual child, many were able to surmount these difficulties and move ahead to normal or superior academic and social achievement. In general, the overall prognostic implications are very encouraging, but the outlook cannot be regarded as uniformly favourable (Menkes, Rowe and Menkes, 1967). The variability in prognosis obviously must depend upon variability in the two underlying features of aetiology and management. Where developmental delay or slow maturation is responsible for a child's motor problems and he is exposed to a satisfactory plan of remediation after early recognition and is of normal or superior intelligence, the prognosis is likely to be excellent. A relatively poor prognosis is augured by an implied organic structural aetiology where late recognition has resulted in early exclusion from educational facilities because of secondary emotional problems that have developed in the child and have an effect on his environment.

Denhoff (1973), in discussing the natural life history of children with minimal brain dysfunction, observed that there was often a changing clinical picture over a 10-year span with diminishing signs of neurological dysfunction and evidence of increasing IQ scores. His long-term, follow-up study suggested that comprehensively treated children with minimal brain dysfunction were found to have much brighter outcomes as adults when psychostimulant medication was part of the therapy. There was no evidence to show that any harmful immediate or long-term effects occurred when such medication was properly prescribed for a specific behavioural syndrome. We are really still in need of further follow-up information before accurate prognostication can be developed in the syndrome of developmental clumsiness. For instance, there is still much to be learned about which signs augur an unfavourable outcome, and which treatment methods are superior.

It is difficult to assess the extent to which developmental clumsiness in children might be an artifact induced by current environmental demands. With an increasing competitiveness of the environment there is likely to be an increasing rate of failure where conceivably not 5 to 10 per cent, but perhaps up to 50 per cent of ordinary children would be regarded as manifesting developmental clumsiness or related neurodevelopmental disorders. One obvious major problem of school assessment is that standardised appraisals must be made when dealing with large numbers of pupils. With considerable individual variations many children might be regarded as abnormal when compared to the average of their peer groups. In fact they may be perfectly normal in terms of the intactness of their own central nervous systems, psychological behaviour and response to learning. When children leave school, primary school in particular, and they are less subjected to comparisons with norms and standards, many previously observed problems are likely to disappear completely. The clumsy adolescent or adult is left to find his own level when he can dispense with artificially created difficulties. Merely by intelligent avoidance or concealment of physical tasks at which he is inept he can obviate these problems of performance. In any case, he would probably never aspire to becoming a dentist, watchmaker, artist or dancer. He might even be far more successful in terms of adjustment, happiness and achievement in business or alternative professions or trades than even his highly dexterous counterpart. In some instances it would be discreet for the medical advisor at the time of school leaving age to give some general vocational guidance. Surely, one of our major responsibilities to children is to facilitate their progress through school in a happy challenging atmosphere where individual subnormalities are fully appreciated, explained and accepted.

References

Abercrombie, M. L. J. (1964) *Perceptual and Visuo-motor Disorders in Cerebral Palsy. Little Club Clinics in Developmental Medicine,* No. 11, pp. 30 and 47. London: Spastics Society.

Abrams, A. L. (1968) Delayed and irregular maturation versus minimal brain injury. Recommendations for a change in current nomenclature. *Clinical Pediatrics,* **7,** 344–349.

Adams, R. D. & Sidman, R. L. (1968) *Introduction to Neuropathology,* p. 248. New York: McGraw-Hill.

Albitreccia, S. I. (1958) Recognition and treatment of disturbances of the body image. *Cerebral Palsy Bulletin,* **1**(4), 12–17.

Albitreccia, S. I. (1959) Treatment of disorders of the body image. *Spastics Quarterly,* **8**(3), 30–32.

Alpers, B. J. & Mancall, E. L. (1971) *Clinical Neurology,* 6th ed., p. 702. Philadelphia: Davis.

Anderson, C. M. (1956) Early brain injury and behaviour. *Journal of the American Medical Women's Association,* **11,** 113–119.

Anderson, C. M. & Plymate, H. B. (1962) Management of the brain-damaged adolescent. *American Journal of Orthopsychiatry,* **32,** 492–500.

Anderson, W. W. (1963) The hyperkinetic child: a neurological appraisal. *Neurology (Minneapolis),* **13,** 968–973.

Andrews, G. & Harris, M. (1964) Stammering. In *The Child Who Does Not Talk* (Ed.) Renfrew, C. & Murphy, K. *Clinics in Developmental Medicine,* No. 13, pp. 184–192. London: Spastics Society.

Annell, A. L. (1949) School problems in children of average or superior intelligence: a preliminary report. *Journal of Mental Science,* **95,** 901–909.

Annett, M., Lee, D. & Ounsted, C. (1961) Intellectual disabilities in relation to lateralised features in the EEG. In *Hemiplegic Cerebral Palsy in Children and Adults. Little Club Clinics in Developmental Medicine,* No. 4, pp. 86–112. London: Spastics Society.

Apgar, V. (1953) A proposal for a new method of evaluation of the newborn infant. *Anesthesia and Analgesia; Current Researches,* **32,** 260–267.

Apgar, V., Girdany, B. R., McIntosh, R. & Taylor, H. C. (1955) I. A study of the relation of oxygenation at birth to intellectual development. *Pediatrics,* **15,** 653–662.

Ayres, A. J. (1964a) *Southern California Figure–Ground Visual Perception Test.* Protocol Booklet. Los Angeles: Western Psychological Services.

Ayres, A. J. (1964b) *Southern California Motor Accuracy Test.* Test Booklet. Los Angeles: Western Psychological Services.

Ayres, A. J. (1966) *Southern California Kinesthesia and Tactile Perception Tests.* Protocol Booklet. Los Angeles: Western Psychological Services.

Ayres, A. J. (1972a) *Sensory Integration and Learning Disorders.* California: Western Psychological Services.

Ayres, A. J. (1972b) Improving academic scores through sensory integration. *Journal of Learning Disabilities,* **5,** 338–343.

Bakwin, H. (1967) Developmental hyperactivity. *Acta Paediatrica Scandinavica. Supplement,* **172,** 25–29.

Bakwin, H. (1968a) Symposium on Developmental Disorders of Motility and Language. Foreword. *Pediatric Clinics of North America,* **15,** 565–567.

177

Bakwin, H. (1968b) Delayed speech. *Pediatric Clinics of North America*, **15**, 627–638.
Bakwin, H. & Bakwin, R. M. (1960) *Clinical Management of Behaviour Disorders in Children*. 2nd ed. Philadelphia: W. B. Saunders.
Baldwin, R. W. & Kenny, T. J. (1966) Medical treatment of behaviour disorders. In *Learning Disorders* (Ed.) Hellmuth, J. Vol. 2. Seattle: Special Child Publications.
Balf, C. L. (1952) Birth injuries in relation to post-natal defects. The paediatric interpretation. *Transactions of the Edinburgh Obstetrical Society Session*, **104**, 62–69.
Barsch, R. H. (1967) Memorandum to Advisory Council Members, Officers and Committee Chairman of the C.E.C. Division for Children with Learning Disabilities. Quoted by Paine (1968).
Bateman, B. D. & Schiefelbusch, R. L. (1969) *Minimal Brain Dysfunction in Children*. N. & S.D.C.P. Monograph, No. 2015, pp. 5–17. Washington: Public Health Service Publication.
Bax, M. & Mac Keith, R. (1963) *Minimal Cerebral Dysfunction. Little Club Clinics in Developmental Medicine*, No. 10. London: Spastics Society.
Bax, M. & MacKeith, R. (1963) *Minimal Cerebral Dysfunction. Little Club Clinics in examination. Lancet*, **ii**, 368–370.
Bender, L. (1958) Problems in conceptualization and communication in children with developmental alexia. In *Psychopathology of Communication* (Ed.) Hoch, P. H. & Zubin, J. pp. 155–176. New York: Grune & Stratton.
Benson, D. F. & Geschwind, N. (1968) Cerebral dominance and its disturbances. *Pediatric Clinics of North America*, **15**, 759–769.
Benton, A. L. (1959) *Right-Left Discrimination and Finger Localization*. New York: Hoeber.
Benton, A. L. (1968) Right-left discrimination. *Pediatric Clinics of North America*, **15**, 747–758.
Benton, A. L. (1973) Minimal brain dysfunction from a neuropsychological point of view. In *Minimal Brain Dysfunction* (Ed.) de la Cruz, F. F., Fox, B. H. & Roberts, R. H. pp. 29–37. New York: New York Academy of Sciences.
Benton, A. L. & Bird, J. W. (1963) The EEG and reading disability. *American Journal of Orthopsychiatry*, **33**, 529–531.
Bergès, J. (1966) Les dyspraxies chez l'enfant de 5 à 15 ans. Diagnostic-conduite à tenir. *Revue de Neuropsychiatrie Infantile et d'Hygiene Mentale de l'Enfance*, **14**, 267–276.
Bergès, J. & Lézine, L. (1965) *The Imitation of Gestures. A Technique for Studying the Body Schema and Praxis of Children Three to Six Years of Age. Clinics in Developmental Medicine*, No. 18. London: Heinemann.
Berko, M. J. (1966) Psychological and linguistic implications of brain damage in children. In *Communication Training in Childhood Brain Damage* (Ed.) Mecham, M. J., Berko, M. J., Berko, F. G. & Palmer, M. F. Springfield: Thomas.
Bickerstaff, E. R. (1964) Aetiology of acute hemiplegia in childhood. *British Medical Journal*, **ii**, 82–87.
Bingley, T. (1958) Mental symptoms in temporal lobe epilepsy and temporal lobe gliomas. *Acta Psychiatrica Scandinavica. Supplement 120*, Vol. **33**.
Block, W. M. (1971) Cerebral dysfunctions, clarification, delineation, classification. *XIII International Congress of Pediatrics*, **3**, 143–148. Vienna: Wiener Medizinische Akademie.
Bortner, M. & Birch, H. G. (1960) Perceptual and perceptual-motor dissociation in brain-damaged patients. *Journal of Nervous and Mental Diseases*, **130**, 49–53.
Bortner, M. & Birch, H. G. (1962) Perceptual and perceptual-motor dissociation in cerebral palsied children. *Journal of Nervous and Mental Diseases*, **134**, 103–108.
Boshes, B. & Myklebust, H. R. (1964) A neurological and behavioural study of children with learning disorders. *Neurology (Minneapolis)*, **14**, 7–12.
Bradley, C. (1937) The behaviour of children receiving benzedrine. *American Journal of Psychiatry*, **94**, 577–585.
Bradley, C. (1957) Characteristics and management of children with behaviour problems associated with organic brain damage. *Pediatric Clinics of North America*, November, 1049–1060.
Brain, W. R. (1961) *Speech Disorders, Aphasia, Apraxia and Agnosia*. London: Butterworths.
Brain, W. R. & Walton, J. N. (1969) *Brain's Diseases of the Nervous System*. 7th ed. p. 566. London: Oxford University Press.

Brenner, M. W. & Gillman, S. (1966) Visuomotor ability in schoolchildren—a survey. *Developmental Medicine and Child Neurology*, **8**, 686–703.

Brenner, M. W. & Gillman, S. (1968) Verbal intelligence, visuomotor ability and school achievement. *British Journal of Educational Psychology*, **38**, 75–78.

Brenner, M. W., Gillman, S. & Farrell, M. F. (1968) Clinical study of eight children with visual dysfunction and educational problems. *Journal of Neurological Sciences*, **6**, 45–61.

Brenner, M. W., Gillman, S., Zangwill, O. L. & Farrel, M. (1967) Visuo-motor disability in schoolchildren. *British Medical Journal*, **iv**, 259–262.

British Medical Journal (1962) Clumsy children. **ii**, 1665.

British Medical Journal (1970) Examining schoolchildren. **iii**, 600.

Chalfant, J. C. & Scheffelin, M. A. (1969) *Central Processing Dysfunctions in Children*. N.I.N.D.S. Monograph No. 9. Bethesda: U.S. Dept. of Health, Education and Welfare.

Chase, P. H. (1973) The effects of intrauterine and postnatal undernutrition on normal brain development. In *Minimal Brain Dysfunction* (Ed.) de la Cruz, F. F., Fox, B. H. & Roberts, R. H. pp. 231–244. New York: New York Academy of Sciences.

Chorost, S. B., Spivack, G. & Levine, M. (1959) Bender Gestalt rotations and EEG abnormalities in children. *Journal of Consulting Psychology*, **23**, 559.

Cizkova, J. (1963) 'Minimal brain damage' in neurohormonal function. In *Minimal Cerebral Palsy* (Ed.) Bax, M. & Mac Keith, R. *Little Club Clinics in Developmental Medicine*, No. 10, pp. 67–71. London: Spastics Society.

Clements, S. D. (1966a) *Minimal Brain Dysfunction in Children*. U.S. Dept. of Health, Education and Welfare. No. 1415. Washington: Public Health Service Publication.

Clements, S. D. (1966b) The child with minimal brain dysfunction. *Journal-Lancet (Minneapolis)*, **86**, 121–123.

Clements, S. D., Lehtinen, L. E. & Lukens, J. E. (1963) *Children with Minimal Brain Injury. A Symposium.* Chicago: National Society for Crippled Children and Adults, Inc.

Clements, S. D. & Peters, J. E. (1962) Minimal brain dysfunctions in the school age child. *Archives of General Psychiatry*, **6**, 185–197.

Clements, S. D. & Peters, J. E. (1973) Psychoeducational programming for children with minimal brain dysfunctions. In *Minimal Brain Dysfunction* (Ed.) de la Cruz, F. F., Fox, B. H. & Roberts, R. H. pp. 46–51. New York: New York Academy of Sciences.

Clemmens, R. L. (1961) Minimal brain damage in children—an interdisciplinary problem, medical, paramedical, and educational. *Children*, **8**, 179–183.

Cohen, S. A. (1973) Minimal brain dysfunction and practical matters such as teaching kids to read. In *Minimal Brain Dysfunction* (Ed.) de la Cruz, F. F., Fox, B. H. & Roberts, R. H. pp. 251–261. New York: New York Academy of Sciences.

Cohn, R. (1961a) Dyscalculia. *Archives of Neurology (Chicago)*, **4**, 301–307.

Cohn, R. (1961b) Delayed acquisition of reading and writing abilities in children. *Archives of Neurology (Chicago)*, **4**, 153–164.

Cohn, R. (1964) The neurological study of children with learning disabilities. *Exceptional Children*, **31**, 179–185.

Cohn, R. (1968) Developmental dyscalculia. *Pediatric Clinics of North America*, **15**, 651–668.

Collier, J. S. Quoted by Ford, F. R. (1966).

Collins, E. & Turner, G. (1971) The importance of the 'small-for-dates' baby to the problem of mental retardation. *Medical Journal of Australia*, **2**, 313–315.

Conners, C. K. (1967) The syndrome of minimal brain dysfunction: psychological aspects. *Pediatric Clinics of North America*, **14**, 749–766.

Conners, C. K. & Eisenberg, L. (1963) The effects of methylphenidate on symptomatology and learning in disturbed children. *American Journal of Psychiatry*, **120**, 458–464.

Connolly, K. (1968) The applications of operant conditioning to the measurement and development of motor skills in children. *Developmental Medicine and Child Neurology*, **10**, 697–705.

Coppele, P. J. & Isom, J. B. (1968) Soft signs in scholastic success. *Neurology (Minneapolis)*, **18**, 304.

Crawford, C. (1960) Report of a family showing 'mirror' movements. *Australasian Annals of Medicine*, **9**, 176–179.

Crichton, J. U., Robertson, A. M., Tredger, E. & Dunn, H. G. (1971) The evaluation of minimal cerebral dysfunction in children of low birth weight. *XIII International Congress of Pediatrics*, **3**, 135–140. Vienna: Wiener Medizinische Akademie.

Critchley, M. (1953) *The Parietal Lobes*. London: Arnold.

Critchley, M. (1967) Some observations upon developmental dyslexia. In *Modern Trends in Neurology*, No. 4 (Ed.) Williams, D. London: Butterworths.

Critchley, M. (1968a) Minor neurologic defects in developmental dyslexia. In *Dyslexia Diagnosis and Treatment of Reading Disorders* (Ed.) Keeney, A. H. & Keeney, V. T. Saint Louis: Mosby.

Critchley, M. (1968b) Topics worthy of research. In *Dyslexia Diagnosis and Treatment of Reading Disorders* (Ed.) Keeney, A. H. & Keeney, V. T. Saint Louis: Mosby.

Critchley, M. (1968c) Developmental dyslexia. *Pediatric Clinics of North America*, **15**, 669–676.

Critchley, M. (1970) *The Dyslexic Child* (2nd ed. of *Developmental Dyslexia*). London: Heinemann.

Crothers, B. & Paine, R. S. (1959) *The Natural History of Cerebral Palsy*. Cambridge, Mass.: Harvard University Press.

Cruikshank, W. M., Bice, H. V. & Wallen, N. E. (with the co-operation of Podesek, E. & Thomas, E. P.) (1957) *Perception and Cerebral Palsy: A Study in Figure Background Relationship*. Syracuse: Syracuse University Press.

Da Costa, M. I. L. (1946) *The Ozeretsky Tests of Motor Proficiency*. A translation from the Portuguese adaptation (Ed.) Doll, E. A. Minneapolis: American Guidance Service Inc.

Dare, M. T. & Gordon, N. (1970) Clumsy children: a disorder of perception and motor organisation. *Developmental Medicine and Child Neurology*, **12**, 178–185.

Daryn, E. (1961) Problems of children with 'diffuse brain damage'. *Archives of General Psychiatry*, **4**, 299–306.

Davidoff, R. A. & Johnson, L. C. (1964) Paroxysmal EEG activity and cognitive-motor performance. *Electroencephalography and Clinical Neurophysiology*, **16**, 343–354.

De Hirsch, K. (1954) Gestalt psychology as applied to language disturbances. *Journal of Nervous and Mental Diseases*, **120**, 257–261.

DeJong, R. N. (1967) *The Neurologic Examination*. 3rd ed. New York: Hoeber.

Delacato, C. H. (1963) *The Diagnosis and Treatment of Speech and Reading Problems*. Springfield: Thomas.

De La Cruz, F. & LaVeck, G. D. (1965) The pediatrician's view of learning disorders. In *Learning Disorders* (Ed.) Hellmuth, J. Vol. 1. Seattle: Special Child Publications.

Denhoff, E. D. (1971) The cerebral minimal syndromes (minimal brain dysfunction syndrome). *XIII International Congress of Pediatrics*, **3**, 63–68. Vienna: Wiener Medizinische Akademie.

Denhoff, E. (1973) The natural life history of children with minimal brain dysfunction. In *Minimal Brain Dysfunction* (Ed.) de la Cruz, F. F., Fox, B. H. & Roberts, R. H. pp. 188–205. New York: New York Academy of Sciences.

Denhoff, E., Laufer, M. W. & Holden, R. H. (1959) The syndromes of cerebral dysfunction. *Journal of the Oklahoma State Medical Association*, **52**, 360–366.

Denhoff, E. & Robinault, I. P. (1960) *Cerebral Palsy and Related Disorders*. New York: McGraw-Hill.

Dennis, W (1941) Infant development under conditions of restricted practice and of minimum social stimulation. *Genetic Psychology Monographs*, **23**, 143–189.

Denny-Brown, D. (1958) The nature of apraxia. *Journal of Nervous and Mental Diseases*, **126**, 9–32.

Denny-Brown, D. (1966) *The Cerebral Control of Movement*. Liverpool: Liverpool University Press.

Developmental Medicine and Child Neurology (1968) The Doman-Delacato Treatment of Neurologically Handicapped Children. **10**, 243–246.

Di Cagno, L. & Ravetto, F. (1967) Disturbi practo-gnosici in bambini con danno cerebrale minimo. *Minerva Pediatrica*, **19**, 348–365.

Doll, E. A. (1951) Neurophrenia. *American Journal of Psychiatry*, **108**, 50–53.

Drew, A. L. (1956) Neurological appraisal of familial congenital word-blindness. *Brain*, **79**, 440–460.

Dunsdon, M. I. (1952) *The Educability of the Cerebral Palsied Child*. London: Newnes.

Edwards, N. (1968) The relationship between physical condition immediately after birth and mental and motor performance at age four. *Genetic Psychology Monographs*, **78**, 257–289.

Eisenberg, L. (1957) The psychiatric implications of brain damage in children. *Psychiatric Quarterly*, **31**, 72–92.

Eisenberg, L. (1959) Office evaluation of specific reading disability in children. *Pediatrics*, **23**, 997–1003.

Eisenberg, L. (1966) The management of the hyperkinetic child. *Developmental Medicine and Child Neurology*, **8**, 593–598.

Elizur, A. (1959) A combined test used for the diagnosis of organic brain condition. *Archives of Neurology and Psychiatry (Chicago)*, **81**, 776–784.

Elliott, F. A. (1971) *Clinical Neurology*. 2nd ed., Ch. 9, p. 186. Philadelphia: W. B. Saunders.

Ellis, E. (1967) *The Physical Management of Developmental Disorders. Clinics in Developmental Medicine*, No. 26. London: Spastics Society.

Fait, H. F. (1972) *Special Physical Education; Adaptive, Corrective, Developmental.* 3rd ed. Ch. 13. Philadelphia: W. B. Saunders.

Falconer, M. A. & Cavanagh, J. B. (1959) Clinico-pathological considerations of temporal lobe epilepsy due to small focal lesions. A study of cases submitted to operation. *Brain*, **82**, 483–504.

Floyer, E. B. (1955) *A Psychological Study of a City's Cerebral Palsied Children.* London: British Council for the Welfare of Spastics.

Ford, F. R. (1966) *Diseases of the Nervous System in Infancy, Childhood and Adolescence.* 5th ed. Springfield: Thomas.

Francis-Williams, J. (1963) Problems of development in children with 'minimal brain damage'. In *Minimal Cerebral Dysfunction* (Ed.) Bax, M. & Mac Keith, R. *Little Club Clinics in Developmental Medicine*, No. 10, pp. 39–45. London: Spastics Society.

Fraser, M. S. & Wilks, J. (1959) The residual effects of neonatal asphyxia. *Journal of Obstetrics and Gynaecology of the British Commonwealth*, **66**, 748–752.

Freeman, R. D. (1967) Controversy over 'patterning' as a treatment for brain damage in children. *Journal of the American Medical Association*, **202**(5), 385–388.

Frostig, M. (1963) Visual perception in the brain-injured child. *American Journal of Orthopsychiatry*, **33**, 665–671.

Frostig, M. (1971) Cerebral minimal syndrome: psychological and educational treatment. *XIII International Congress of Pediatrics*, **3**, 11–28. Vienna: Wiener Medizinische Akademie.

Gallagher, J. R. (1960) Specific language disability (dyslexia). *Clinical Proceedings—Children's Hospital Washington D.C.*, **16**, 3–15.

Gallagher, J. J., Kunstadter, R. H., Cole, C. H. & Clements, S. D. (1969) *Minimal Brain Dysfunction in Children.* N. & S.D.C.P. Monograph. No. 2015. Washington: Public Health Service Publication.

Gerstmann, J. (1924) Fingeragnosie. Eine umschriebene Störung der Orientierung am eigenen Körper. *Wiener klinische Wochenschrift*, **37**, 1010–1012.

Gerstmann, J. (1927) Fingeragnosie und isolierte Agraphie—ein neues Syndrom. *Zentralblatt für die gesamte Neurologie und Psychiatrie*, **108**, 152–177.

Gerstmann, J. (1940) Syndrome of finger agnosia, disorientation for right and left, agraphia and acalculia; local diagnostic values. *Archives of Neurology and Psychiatry (Chicago)*, **44**, 398–408.

Geschwind, N. (1965) Disconnection syndromes in animals and man. Part II. *Brain*, **88**, 585–644.

Geschwind, N. (1967) Brain mechanisms suggested by studies of hemispheric connections. In *Brain Mechanisms Underlying Speech and Language* (Ed.) Millikan, C. H. & Darley, F. L. New York: Grune & Stratton.

Gesell, A. L. & Amatruda, C. S. (1947) *Developmental Diagnosis; Normal and Abnormal Child Development; Clinical Methods and Pediatric Applications.* 2nd ed. New York: Hoeber.

Glaser, G. H. (1963) The normal electroencephalogram and its reactivity. *EEG and Behaviour.* Ch. 1, pp. 3–23. New York: Basic Books.

Goldberg, H. K., Marshall, C. & Sims, E. (1960) The role of brain damage in congenital dyslexia. *American Journal of Ophthalmology*, **50**, 586–590.

Gomez, M. R. (1967) Minimal cerebral dysfunction (maximal neurologic confusion). *Clinical Pediatrics (Philadelphia)*, **6**, 589–591.

Gooddy, W. & Reinhold, M. (1961) Congenital dyslexia and asymmetry of cerebral function. *Brain*, **84**, 231–242.

Goodglass, H. & Quadfasel, F. A. (1954) Language laterality in left-handed aphasics. *Brain,* **77,** 521–548.

Gubbay, S. S. (1972) *The Clumsy Child: A Study of Developmental Apraxia and Agnosia.* Thesis for Doctor of Medicine, University of Western Australia.

Gubbay, S. S. (1973) A standardized test battery for the assessment of clumsy children. *Proceedings of the Australian Association of Neurologists,* **10,** 19–25.

Gubbay, S. S. (1975) Clumsy children in normal schools. *Medical Journal of Australia,* **1,** 233–236.

Gubbay, S. S. & Stenhouse, N. S. (1973) Clumsy children: a pilot survey of developmental clumsiness in Western Australia. *Neurology (India) Proceedings, Supplement III,* 454–462.

Gubbay, S. S., Ellis, E., Walton, J. N. & Court, S. D. M. (1965) Clumsy children: a study of apraxic and agnostic defects in 21 children. *Brain,* **88,** 295–312.

Gubbay, S. S., Lobascher, M. & Kingerlee, P. (1970a) A neurological appraisal of autistic children: results of a Western Australian survey. *Developmental Medicine and Child Neurology,* **12,** 422–429.

Gubbay, S. S., Lobascher, M. & Kingerlee, P. (1970b) A neurological appraisal of autistic children: results of a Western Australian Survey. *Proceedings of the Australian Association of Neurologists,* **7,** 103–109.

Gutelius, M. F. & Layman, E. M. (1960) Reading disability of developmental dyslexia. *Clinical Proceedings—Children's Hospital (Washington D.C.),* **16,** 15–27.

Hagberg, B. (1962) The sequelae of spontaneously arrested infantile hydrocephalus. *Developmental Medicine and Child Neurology,* **4,** 583–587.

Hagberg, B. (1963) Minimal brain damage in spontaneously arrested infantile hydrocephalus. In *Minimal Cerebral Dysfunction* (Ed.) Bax, M. & Mac Keith, R. *Little Club Clinics in Developmental Medicine,* No. 10, p. 28. London: Spastics Society.

Hallgren, B. (1950) Specific dyslexia ('congenital word blindness') a clinical and genetic study. *Acta Psychiatrica et Neurologica Scandinavica, Supplement,* **65,** 1–287.

Hansen, E. (1963) Reading and writing difficulties in children with cerebral palsy. In *Minimal Cerebral Dysfunction* (Ed.) Bax, M. & Mac Keith, R. *Little Club Clinics in Developmental Medicine,* No. 10, pp. 58–61. London: Spastics Society.

Hanvick, L. J. (1953) A note on rotations in the Bender Gestalt Test as predictors of EEG abnormalities in children. *Journal of Clinical Psychology,* **9,** 399.

Haring, N. G. (1969) Editor, *Minimal Brain Dysfunction in Children.* N. & S.D.C.P. Monograph. No. 2015. Washington: Public Health Service Publication.

Haring, N. G. & Bateman, B. D. (1969) Introduction. In *Minimal Brain Dysfunction in Children.* N. & S.D.C.P. Monograph. No. 2015, pp. 1–4. Washington: Public Health Service Publication.

Haring, N. G., Reid, W. R. & Beaber, J. D. (1969) Professional preparation for the education of children with learning disabilities. In *Minimal Brain Dysfunction in Children.* N. & S. D. C. P. Monograph. No. 2015, pp. 31–43. Washington: Public Health Service Publication.

Harlow, H. F. & Harlow, M. K. (1962) Principles of primate learning. In *Lessons in Animal Behaviour for the Clinician* (Ed.) Barnett, S. A. *Little Club Clinics in Developmental Medicine,* No. 7., pp 33–48. London: Spastics Society.

Hatton, D. A. (1966) The child with minimal cerebral dysfunction; a child guidance clinic's approach to diagnosis and treatment. *Developmental Medicine and Child Neurology,* **8,** 71–78.

Hawke, W. A. (1971) A critical look at methods of assessment and remediation. *XIII International Congress of Pediatrics,* **3,** 115–120. Vienna: Wiener Medizinische Akademie.

Hécaen, H. (1967) Brain mechanisms suggested by studies of parietal lobes. In *Brain Mechanisms Underlying Speech and Language* (Ed.) Millikan, C. H. & Darley, F. L. New York: Grune & Stratton.

Heilman, K. M. (1973) Ideational apraxia—a re-definition. *Brain,* **96,** 861–864.

Hermann, K. (1956) Congenital word-blindness (poor readers in the light of Gerstmann's Syndrome). *Acta Psychiatrica Scandinavica Supplement (Kobenhaven),* **108,** 177–184.

Hermann, K. & Norrie, E. (1958) Is congenital word-blindness a hereditary type of Gerstmann's syndrome? *Psychiatria et Neurologia (Basel),* **136,** 59–73.

Illingworth, R. S. (1963) The clumsy child. In *Minimal Cerebral Dysfunction* (Ed.) Bax, M. &

Mac Keith, R. *Little Club Clinics in Developmental Medicine*, No. 10, pp. 26–27. London: Spastics Society.

Illingworth, R. S. (1968) Delayed motor development. *Pediatric Clinics of North America*, **15**, 569–580.

Illingworth, R. S. (1971) Prenatal, perinatal and postnatal factors affecting psychological development of the child. *XIII International Congress of Pediatrics*, **3**, 1–8. Vienna: Wiener Medizinische Akademie.

Ingram, T. T. S. (1956) A characteristic form of overactive behaviour in brain damaged children. *Journal of Mental Science*, **102**, 550–558.

Ingram, T. T. S. (1960) Perceptual disorders causing dyslexia and dysgraphia in cerebral palsy. In *Child Neurology and Cerebral Palsy* (Ed.) Bax, M., Clayton-Jones, E. & Mac Keith, R. *Little Club Clinics in Developmental Medicine*, No. 2, pp. 97–104. London: Spastics Society.

Ingram, T. T. S. (1963) Chronic brain syndromes in childhood other than cerebral palsy, epilepsy and mental defect. In *Minimal Cerebral Dysfunction* (Ed.) Bax, M. & Mac Keith, R. *Little Club Clinics in Developmental Medicine*, No. 10, pp. 10–17. London: Spastics Society.

Ingram, T. (1964) The complex speech disorders of cerebral palsied children. In *The Child Who Does Not Talk* (Ed.) Renfrew, C. & Murphy, K. *Clinics in Developmental Medicine*, No. 13, pp. 163–167. London: Spastics Society.

Ingram, T. T. S. (1968) Speech disorders in childhood. *Pediatric Clinics of North America*, **15**, 611–626.

Ingram, T. T. S. (1973) Soft signs. *Developmental Medicine and Child Neurology*, **15**, 527–530.

Isom, J. B. (1966) Perceptual development: visual and kinesthetic. A brief review. *Physical Therapy*, **46**, 734–740.

James, C. C. M. & Lassman, L. P. (1967) Results of treatment of progressive lesions in spina bifida occulta five to ten years after laminectomy. *Lancet*, **ii**, 1277–1279.

Jasper, H. H. & Raney, E. T. (1937) The phi test of lateral dominance. *American Journal of Psychology*, **49**, 450–457.

Kahn, E. & Cohen, L. H. (1934) Organic driveness, a brain-stem syndrome and an experience. With case reports. *New England Journal of Medicine*, **210**, 748–756.

Kalverboer, A. F., Touwen, B. C. L. & Prechtl, H. F. R. (1973) Follow-up of infants at risk of minor brain dysfunction. In *Minimal Brain Dysfunction* (Ed.) de la Cruz, F. F., Fox, B. H. & Roberts, R. H., pp. 173–187. New York: New York Academy of Sciences.

Kass, C. E., Hall, R. E. & Simches, R. F. (1969) Legislation in minimal brain dysfunction in children. In *Minimal Brain Dysfunction in Children*. N. & S.D.C.P. Monograph No. 2015, pp. 44–50. Washington: Public Health Service Publication.

Kawi, A. A. & Pasamanick, B. (1958) Association of factors of pregnancy with reading disorders in childhood. *Journal of the American Medical Association*, **166**, 1420–1423.

Kennard, M. A. (1960) Value of equivocal signs in neurological diagnosis. *Neurology (Minneapolis)*, **10**, 753–764.

Kephart, N. C. (1971) *The Slow Learner in the Classroom*. 2nd ed. Columbus: Merrill.

Kerr, J. (1897) School hygiene in its mental, moral and physical aspects. *Journal of the Royal Statistical Society*, **60**, 613–680.

Kiloh, L. G. & Osselton, J. Q. (1961) *Clinical Electroencephalography*, pp. 101–102. London: Butterworths.

Kinsbourne, M. (1968) Developmental Gerstmann syndrome. *Pediatric Clinics of North America*, **15**, 771–778.

Kinsbourne, M. (1973) Minimal brain dysfunction as a neurodevelopmental lag. In *Minimal Brain Dysfunction* (Ed.) de la Cruz, F. F., Fox, B. H. & Roberts, R. H., pp. 268–273. New York: New York Academy of Sciences.

Kinsbourne, M. & Warrington, E. K. (1962) A study of finger agnosia. *Brain*, **85**, 47–66.

Kinsbourne, M. & Warrington, E. K. (1963a) The relevance of delayed acquisition of finger sense to backwardness in reading and writing. In *Minimal Cerebral Dysfunction* (Ed.) Bax, M. & Mac Keith, R. *Little Club Clinics in Developmental Medicine*, No. 10, pp. 62–64. London: Spastics Society.

Kinsbourne, M. & Warrington, E. K. (1963b) A survey of finger sense among retarded readers. In *Minimal Cerebral Dysfunction* (Ed.) Bax, M. & Mac Keith, R. *Little Club Clinics in Developmental Medicine*, No. 10, pp. 65–66. London: Spastics Society.

Kirk, S. A. (1968) Illinois test of psycholinguistic abilities: Its origins and implications. In *Learning Disorders* (Ed.) Hellmuth, J. Vol. 3. Seattle: Special Child Publications.

Klapper, Z. S. (1966) Reading retardation: II. Psychoeducational aspects of reading disabilities. *Pediatrics,* **37,** 366–376.

Klasen, E. (1972) *The Syndrome of Specific Dyslexia.* Lancaster: MTP.

Knight, J. A., McGovern, J. P., Haywood, T. J. & Chao, D. H. (1962) Headaches in children: II. The psychological implications of headache in children. *Headache,* **1,** 30–37.

Knobloch, H. & Pasamanick, B. (1959) Syndrome of minimal cerebral damage in infancy. *Journal of the American Medical Association,* **170,** 1384–1387.

Köng, E. (1963) Minimal cerebral palsy: the importance of its recognition. In *Minimal Cerebral Dysfunction* (Ed.) Bax, M. & Mac Keith, R. *Little Club Clinics in Developmental Medicine,* No. 10, pp. 29–31. London: Spastics Society.

Kramer, F. & Pollnow, H. (1932) Uber eine hyperkinetische Erkrankung im Kindesalter. *Monatsschrift für Psychiatrie und Neurologie,* **82,** 1–40.

Langworthy, O. R. (1970) *The Sensory Control of Posture and Movement—A Review of the Studies of Derek Denny-Brown.* Baltimore: Williams & Wilkins.

Lilienfeld, A. M. & Pasamanick, B. (1954) Association of maternal and fetal factors with the development of epilepsy. I: Abnormalities in the prenatal and paranatal periods. *Journal of the American Medical Association,* **155,** 719–724.

Lilienfeld, A. M. & Pasamanick, B. (1955) The association of maternal and fetal factors with the development of cerebral palsy and epilepsy. *American Journal of Obstetrics and Gynecology,* **70,** 93–101.

Lissauer, H. (1889) Ein Fall von Seelenblindheit nebst einem Beitrage zur Theorie derselben. *Archiv für Psychiatrie und Nervenkrankheiten,* **21,** 222–270.

Lobascher, M. E., Kingerlee, P. E. & Gubbay, S. S. (1970) Childhood autism: an investigation of aetiological factors in twenty-five cases. *British Journal of Psychiatry,* **117,** 525–529.

Lord, E. E. (1937) *Children Handicapped by Cerebral Palsy. Psychological Factors in Management.* New York: The Commonwealth Fund.

Lucas, A. R., Rodin, E. A. & Simson, C. B. (1965) Neurological assessment of children with early school problems. *Developmental Medicine and Child Neurology,* **7,** 145–156.

Luria, A. R. (1966) *Higher Cortical Functions in Man.* New York: Basic Books.

Mc.Aninch, M. (1966) Body image as related to perceptual-cognitive-motor disabilities. In *Learning Disorders* (Ed.) Hellmuth, J. Vol. 2. Seattle: Special Child Publications.

McFie, J. (1952) Cerebral dominance in cases of reading disability. *Journal of Neurology, Neurosurgery and Psychiatry,* **15,** 194–199.

McFie, J. (1963) An introduction to the problem of 'minimal brain damage'. In *Minimal Cerebral Dysfunction* (Ed.) Bax, M. & Mac Keith, R. *Little Club Clinics in Developmental Medicine,* No. 10, pp. 18–23. London: Spastics Society.

McFie, J., Piercy, M. F. & Zangwill, O. L. (1950) Visual-spatial agnosia associated with lesions of the right cerebral hemisphere. *Brain,* **73,** 167–189.

McFie, J. & Zangwill, O. L. (1960) Visual-constructive disabilities associated with lesions of the left cerebral hemisphere. *Brain,* **83,** 243–259.

MacKeith, R. (1963) Defining the concept of 'minimal brain damage'. In *Minimal Cerebral Dysfunction* (Ed.) Bax, M. & Mac Keith, R. *Little Club Clinics in Developmental Medicine,* No. 10, pp. 1–9. London: Spastics Society.

MacKeith, R. C. (1968) Maximal clarity on neurodevelopmental disorders. *Developmental Medicine and Child Neurology,* **10,** 143–144.

Mark, H. J. (1969) Psychodiagnostics in patients with suspected minimal brain dysfunctions. In *Minimal Brain Dysfunction in Children.* N. & S.D.C.P. Monograph. No. 2015, pp. 72–81. Washington: Public Health Service Publication.

Masland, R. L. (1969a) Preface. In *Central Processing Dysfunction in Children* (Ed.) Chalfant, J. C. & Scheffelin, M. A. N.I.N.D.S. Monograph. No. 9. Washington: U.S. Dept. Of Health Education and Welfare.

Masland, R. L. (1969b) Summary and Reflections. In *Perceptual-Motor Foundations: A Multidisciplinary Approach* (Ed.) Sloan, M. R., Jones, A. W. & Misner, D. E., pp. 155–163. Washington: Association for Health, Physical Education and Recreation.

Masland, R. L. (1973) Epilogue. In *Minimal Brain Dysfunction* (Ed.) de la Cruz, F. F., Fox, B. H. & Roberts, R. H., pp. 395–396. New York: New York Academy of Sciences.

Medical Journal of Australia (1971) The small-for-dates baby. **2,** 291–292.

Menkes, M. M., Rowe, J. S. & Menkes, J. H. (1967) A twenty-five year follow-up study on the hyperkinetic child with minimal brain dysfunction. *Pediatrics*, **39**, 393–399.

Michel, G. (1963) Notes on the so-called 'minimal brain damage' syndrome with particular reference to family dynamics. In *Minimal Cerebral Dysfunction* (Ed.) Bax, M. & Mac Keith, R. *Little Club Clinics in Developmental Medicine*, No. 10, pp. 52–57. London: Spastics Society.

Miller, C. A. (1969) Minimal brain dysfunction—National project on learning disabilities in children. Report of Committee on medical and health-related services. In *Minimal Brain Dysfunction in Children*. N. & S.D.C.P. Monograph. No. 2015, pp. 51–81. Washington: Public Health Service Publication.

Millichap, J. G. (1968) Drugs in management of hyperkinetic and perceptually handicapped children. *Journal of the American Medical Association*, **206**, 1527–1530.

Millichap, J. G. (1973) Drugs in management of minimal brain dysfunction. In *Minimal Brain Dysfunction* (Ed.) de la Cruz, F. F., Fox, B. H. & Roberts, R. H., pp. 321–334. New York: New York Academy of Sciences.

Millichap, J. G., Aymat, F., Sturgis, L. H., Larsen, K. W. & Egan, R. A. (1968) Hyperkinetic behaviour and learning disorders. III. Battery of neuropsychological tests in controlled trial of methylphenidate. *American Journal of Diseases of Children*, **116**, 235–244.

Millichap, J. G. & Boldrey, E. E. (1967) Studies in hyperkinetic behaviour. II. Laboratory and clinical evaluations of drug treatments. *Neurology (Minneapolis)*, **17**, 467–471.

Millichap, J. G. & Fowler, G. W. (1967) Treatment of 'minimal brain dysfunction' syndromes. Selection of drugs for children with hyperactivity and learning disorders. *Pediatric Clinics of North America*, **14**, 767–777.

Minskoff, J. G. (1973) Differential approaches to prevalence estimates of learning disabilities. In *Minimal Brain Dysfunction* (Ed.) de la Cruz, F. F., Fox, B. H. & Roberts, R. H. pp. 139–145. New York: New York Academy of Sciences.

Morgan, W. P. (1896) A case of congenital word blindness. *British Medical Journal*, **ii**, 1378.

Morley, M. E. (1957) *The Development and Disorders of Speech in Childhood*. Edinburgh: Livingstone.

Morley, M., Court, D. & Miller, H. (1954) Developmental dysarthria. *British Medical Journal*, **i**, 8–10.

Morley, M., Court, D., Miller, H. & Garside, R. F. (1955) Delayed speech and developmental aphasia. *British Medical Journal*, **ii**, 463–467.

Morris, P. R. & Whiting, H. T. A. (1971) *Motor Impairment and Compensatory Education*. Ch. 7. London: Bell.

National Advisory Committee on Handicapped Children (1967) Conference sponsored by Bureau of Education for the Handicapped. U.S. Office of Education, Washington, D.C. 1967.

Needleman, H. L. (1973) Lead poisoning in children: Neurologic implications of widespread subclinical intoxication. In *Minimal Cerebral Dysfunction in Children* (Ed.) Walzer, S. & Wolff, P. H. pp. 47–54. New York: Grune & Stratton.

Nielsen, J. M. (1962) *Agnosia, Apraxia, Aphasia. Their Value in Cerebral Localisation*. 2nd ed. New York: Hafner.

Omenn, G. S. (1973) Genetic issues in the syndrome of minimal brain dysfunction. In *Minimal Cerebral Dysfunction in Children* (Ed.) Walzer, S. & Wolff, P. H. pp. 5–17. New York: Grune & Stratton.

Orton, S. T. (1937) *Reading Writing and Speech Problems in Children*. New York: Norton.

Ounsted, C. (1955) The hyperkinetic syndrome in epileptic children. *Lancet*, **ii**, 303–311.

Ozer, M. N. (1968) The neurological evaluation of school-age children. *Journal of Learning Disabilities*, **1**(1), 84–88.

Ozer, M. N. & Richardson, H. B. (1969) Standardised motor examination of pre-school children as a predictor of school performance. *Developmental Medicine and Child Neurology*, **11**, 251.

Ozeretsky, N. (see Da Costa, 1946).

Paine, R. S. (1962) Minimal chronic brain syndromes in children. *Developmental Medicine and Child Neurology*, **4**, 21–27.

Paine, R. S. (1965) Organic neurological factors related to learning disorders. In *Learning Disorders* (Ed.) Hellmuth, J. Seattle: Special Child Publications.

Paine, R. S. (1968) Syndromes of 'minimal cerebral damage'. *Pediatric Clinics of North America*, **15**, 779–801.

Paine, R. S. & Oppé, T. E. (1966) Neurological examination of children. *Clinics in Developmental Medicine*, Nos. 21 & 22. London: Spastics Society.

Paine, R. S., Werry, J. S. & Quay, H. C. (1968) A study of 'minimal cerebral dysfunction'. *Developmental Medicine and Child Neurology*, **10,** 505–520.

Pasamanick, B. & Kawi, A. (1956) A study of the association of prenatal and paranatal factors with the development of tics in children: a preliminary investigation. *Journal of Pediatrics,* **48,** 596–601.

Pasamanick, B. & Lilienfeld, A. M. (1955) Association of maternal and fetal factors with development of mental deficiency. I. Abnormalities in the prenatal and paranatal periods. *Journal of the American Medical Association,* **159,** 155–160.

Pincus, J. H. & Glaser, G. H. (1966) The syndrome of 'minimal brain damage' in childhood. *New England Journal of Medicine,* **275,** 27–35.

Pond, D. (1960) Is there a syndrome of 'brain damage' in children? *Cerebral Palsy Bulletin,* **2,** 296–297.

Pond, D. A. (1961) Psychiatric aspects of epileptic and brain-damaged children. *British Medical Journal,* **ii,** 1377–1382.

Pratt, R. T. C. (1967) *The Genetics of Neurological Disorders.* p. 127. London: Oxford University Press.

Prechtl, H. F. R. (1960) The long term value of the neurological examination of the newborn infant. In *Child Neurology and Cerebral Palsy. Little Club Clinics in Developmental Medicine,* No. 2, pp. 69–74. London: Spastics Society.

Prechtl, H. F. R. & Stemmer, J. C. (1962) The choreiform syndrome in children. *Developmental Medicine and Child Neurology,* **4,** 119–127.

Rabe, E. F. (1969) Neurological evaluation. In *Minimal Brain Dysfunction in Children.* N. & S. D. C. P. Monograph. No. 2015, pp. 69–71. Washington: Public Health Service Publication.

Rabinovich, R. D., Drew, A. L., DeJong, R. N., Ingram, W. & Withey, L. (1954) A research approach to reading retardation. In *Neurology and Psychiatry in Childhood. Research Publications of the Association for Research in Nervous and Mental Disease,* **34,** 363–396.

Reuben, R. N. & Bakwin, H. (1968) Developmental clumsiness. *Pediatric Clinics of North America,* **15,** 601–610.

Robbins, M. P. (1967) Test of the Doman-Delacato rationale with retarded readers. *Journal of the American Medical Association,* **202**(5), 389–393.

Rodin, E., Lucas, A. & Simon, C. (1964) A study of behaviour disorders in children by means of general purpose computers. *Data Acquisition and Processing in Biology and Medicine,* **3,** 115–124.

Rogan, L. L. & Lukens, J. E. (1969) Education, administration and classroom procedures. In *Minimal Brain Dysfunction in Children.* N. & S.D.C.P. Monograph, No. 2015, pp. 21–30. Washington: Public Health Service Publication.

Rogers, M. E., Lilienfeld, A. M. & Pasamanick, B. (1955) Prenatal and paranatal factors in the development of childhood behaviour disorders. *Acta Psychiatrica et Neurologica Scandinavica Supplement,* **102,** 1–157.

Russell, W. R. (1960) The parietal lobes. In *Child Neurology and Cerebral Palsy* (Ed.) Bax, M., Clayton-Jones, E. & Mac Keith, R. *Little Club Clinics in Developmental Medicine,* No. 2, pp. 110–114. London: Spastics Society.

Rutter, M., Graham, P. & Birch, H. G. (1966) Interrelations between the choreiform syndrome, reading disability and psychiatric disorder in children of 8–11 years. *Developmental Medicine and Child Neurology,* **8,** 149–159.

Rutter, M., Tizard, J. & Whitmore, K. (1970) *Education Health and Behaviour.* Psychological and Medical Study of Childhood Development. London: Longman.

Satterfield, J. H. (1973) EEG issues in children with minimal brain dysfunction. In *Minimal Cerebral Dysfunction in Children* (Ed.) Walzer, S. & Wolff, P. H., pp. 35–46. New York: Grune & Stratton.

Satterfield, J. H., Lesser, L. I., Saul, R. E. & Cantwell, D. P. (1973) EEG aspects in the diagnosis and treatment of children with minimal brain dysfunction. In *Minimal Brain Dysfunction* (Ed.) de la Cruz, F. F., Fox, B. H. & Roberts, R. H. New York: New York Academy of Sciences.

Schain, R. J. (1972) *Neurology of Childhood Learning Disorders.* Baltimore: Williams & Wilkins.

Schiller, F. (1969) Dysarthria, aphasia and apraxia. In *Bing's Local Diagnosis in Neurological Diseases* (Ed.) Haymaker, W. p. 402. Saint Louis: Mosby.

Schonell, F. J. & Schonell, F. E. (1950) *Diagnostic and Attainment Testing.* Edinburgh: Oliver & Boyd.

Sechzer, J. A., Faro, M. D. & Windle, W. F. (1973) Studies of monkeys asphyxiated at birth: Implications for minimal cerebral dysfunction. In *Minimal Cerebral Dysfunction in Children* (Ed.) Walzer, S. & Wolff, P. H., pp. 19–34. New York: Grune & Stratton.

Silverman, L. J. & Metz, A. S. (1973) Numbers of pupils with specific learning disabilities in local public schools in the United States. In *Minimal Brain Dysfunction* (Ed.) de la Cruz, F. F., Fox, B. H. & Roberts, R. H., pp. 146–157. New York: New York Academy of Sciences.

Skatvedt, M. (1960) Sensory, perceptual and other non-motor defects in cerebral palsy. In *Child Neurology and Cerebral Palsy* (Ed.) Bax, M., Clayton-Jones, E. & Mac Keith, R. *Little Club Clinics in Developmental Medicine,* No.2, pp. 115–119. London: Spastics Society.

Skatvedt, M. (1963) Minimal brain damage. In *Minimal Cerebral Dysfunction* (Ed.) Bax, M. & Mac Keith, R. *Little Club Clinics in Developmental Medicine,* No. 10, pp. 32–33. London: Spastics Society.

Snyder, S. H. & Meyerhoff, J. L. (1973) How amphetamine acts in minimal brain dysfunction. In *Minimal Brain Dysfunction* (Ed.) de la Cruz, F. F., Fox, B. H. & Roberts, R. H., pp. 310–320, New York: New York Academy of Sciences.

Solomons, G. (1973) Drug therapy: initiation and follow-up. In *Minimal Brain Dysfunction* (Ed.) de la Cruz, F. F., Fox, B. H. & Roberts, R. H., pp. 335–344. New York: New York Academy of Sciences.

Spillane, J. D. (1942) Disturbances of the body scheme, anosognosia and finger agnosia. *Lancet,* **i,** 42–44.

Stambak, M., L'Heriteau, D., Auzias, M., Bèrges, J. & Ajuriaguerra, J. (1964) Les dyspraxies chez l'enfant. *La Psychoogie de l'Enfant,* **7,** 381–496.

Steckler, G. (1964) A longitudinal follow-up of neonatal apnea. *Child Development,* **35,** 333–348.

Stein, J. U. (1971) Perceptual-motor development of handicapped children—thoughts, observations and questions. In *Foundations and Practices in Perceptual Motor Learning—A Quest for Understanding,* pp. 28–31. Washington: American Association for Health, Physical Health and Recreation.

Stemmer, J. C. (1964) *Choreatiforme Bewegungsonrust.* University of Groningen doctoral thesis. Quoted by Rutter, Graham &Birch (1966).

Stevens, G. D. & Birch, J. W. (1957) A proposal for clarification of the terminology used to describe brain-injured children. *Exceptional Children,* **23,** 346–349.

Stott, D. H. (1957) Physical and mental handicaps following a disturbed pregnancy. *Lancet,* **i,** 1006–1012.

Stott, D. H. (1966) A general test of motor impairment for children. *Developmental Medicine and Child Neurology,* **8,** 523–531.

Stott, D. H., Moyes, F. A. & Headridge, S. E. (1970) *Tests of Motor Impairment* (derived from the Göllnitz revision of the Oseretzky test of motor ability) 4th revision. University of Guelph, Guelph, Ontario, in preparation.

Strauss, A. A. & Lehtinen, C. E. (1947) *Psychopathology and Education of the Brain-Injured Child.* New York: Grune & Stratton.

Strauss, A. A. & Werner, H. (1942) Disorders of conceptual thinking in the brain-injured child. *Journal of Nervous and Mental Disease,* **96,** 153–172.

Strother, C. R. (1973) Minimal cerebral dysfunction: a historical overview. In *Minimal Brain Dysfunction* (Ed.) de la Cruz, F. F., Fox, B. H. & Roberts, R. H., pp. 6–17. New York: New York Academy of Sciences.

Taylor, E. M. (1959) *Psychological Appraisal of Children with Cerebral Defects.* Cambridge, Mass.: Harvard University Press.

Teuber, H. L. & Rudel, R. G. (1962) Behaviour after cerebral lesions in children and adults. *Developmental Medicine and Child Neurology,* **4,** 3–20.

Thelander, H. E., Phelps, J. K. & Kirk, E. W. (1958) Learning disabilities associated with lesser brain damage. *Journal of Pediatrics,* **53,** 405–409.

Thetford, W. N., Schulman, H. & Farmer, C. (1967) Psychological testing of children afflicted with headaches. In *Headaches in Children* (Ed.) Friedman, A. P. & Harms, E. Springfield:

Thomas.

Timme, A. R. (1948) The choreiform syndrome; its significance in children's behaviour. *California Medicine,* **68,** 154–158.

Touwen, B. C. L. & Prechtl, H. F. R. (1970) *The Neurological Examination of the Child with Minor Nervous Dysfunction. Clinics in Developmental Medicine,* No. 38. London: Spastics International.

Twitchell, T. E., Lecours, A. R., Rudel, R. G. & Teuber, H. L. (1966) Minimal cerebral dysfunction in children: Motor deficits. *Transactions of the American Neurological Association,* **91,** 353–355.

Wallon, H. & Denjean, G. (1958) Sur quelques signes d'apraxie chez des enfants 'inadeptés'. *Annales Médico-Psychologiques,* **2,** 1–14.

Walshe, F. M. R. (1965) *Further Critical Studies in Neurology and Other Essays and Addresses.* Edinburgh: Livingstone.

Walton, J. N. (1956) Amyotonia congenita. A follow-up study. *Lancet,* **i,** 1023–1023.

Walton, J. N. (1961) Clumsy children. *Spastics Quarterly,* **10,** 9–21.

Walton, J. N. (1963) Clumsy children. In *Minimal Cerebral Dysfunction* (Ed.) Bax, M. & Mac Keith, R. *Little Club Clinics in Developmental Medicine,* No. 10, pp. 24–25. London: Spastics Society.

Walton, J. N. (1966) *Essentials of Neurology.* 2nd ed. London: Pitman.

Walton, J. N., Ellis, E. & Court, S. D. M. (1962) Clumsy children: a study of developmental apraxia and agnosia. *Brain,* **85,** 603–612.

Walzer, S. & Richmond, J. B. (1973) Introduction. In *Minimal Cerebral Dysfunction in Children* (Ed.) Walzer, S. & Wolff, P. H., pp. 1–3, New York: Grune & Stratton.

Wedell, K. (1961). Follow-up study of perceptual ability in children with hemiplegia. In *Hemiplegic Cerebral Palsy in Children and Adults,* No. 4, pp. 76–83. London: Spastics Society.

Wenar, C. (1963) The reliability of developmental histories. *Psychosomatic Medicine,* **25,** 505–509.

Wender, P. H. (1971) *Minimal Brain Dysfunction in Children.* New York: Wiley-Interscience.

Wender, P. H. (1973) Some speculations concerning a possible biochemical basis of minimal brain dysfunction. In *Minimal Brain Dysfunction* (Ed.) de la Cruz, F. F., Fox, B. H. & Roberts, R. H., pp. 18–28. New York: New York Academy of Sciences.

Werner, H. & Kaplan, B. (1963) *Symbol Formation.* New York: Wiley.

Wernicke, K. (1874) *Der aphasische Symptomencomplex: Eine psychologische Studie auf anatomischer Basis.* Breslau: Cohn und Weigert.

Werry, J. S. (1968) Developmental hyperactivity. *Pediatric Clinics of North America,* **15,** 581–599.

Wigglesworth, R. (1961) Minimal cerebral palsy. *Cerebral Palsy Bulletin,* **3,** 293–295.

Wigglesworth, R. (1963) The importance of recognising minimal cerebral dysfunction in pediatric practice. In *Minimal Cerebral Dysfunction* (Ed.) Bax, M. & Mac Keith, R. *Little Club Clinics in Developmental Medicine,* No. 10, pp. 34–38. London: Spastics Society.

Williams, J. (1961) Some perceptual disorders in children with hemiplegia. In *Hemiplegic Cerebral Palsy in Children and Adults* (Ed.) Bax, M. *Little Club Clinics in Developmental Medicine.* No. 4, pp 71–75. London: Spastics Society.

Wolff, S. (1969) *Children Under Stress.* London: Lane.

Wolff, P. H. & Hurwitz, I. (1966) The choreiform syndrome. *Developmental Medicine and Child Neurology,* **4,** 160–165.

Wolff, P. H. & Hurwitz, I. (1973) Functional implications of the minimal brain damage syndrome. In *Minimal Cerebral Dysfunction in Children* (Ed.) Walzer, S. & Wolff, P. H. pp. 105–115. New York: Grune & Stratton.

Wolfik, D. (1973) Minimal brain dysfunction—an approach to treatment. *Medical Journal of Australia,* **2,** 601–605.

Woods, G. E. (1957) *Cerebral Palsy in Childhood; (The Aetiology and Clinical Assessment with Particular Reference to the Findings in Bristol).* Bristol: Wright.

World Health Organisation Technical Report Series, No. 217 (1961).

Yakovlev, P. I. (1947) Paraplegias of hydrocephalics. *American Journal of Mental Deficiency,* **51,** 561–576.

Yates, A. J. (1966) Psychological deficit. *Annual Review of Psychology,* **17,** 111–144.

Zangwill, O. L. (1960a) Deficiency of spatial perception. In *Child Neurology and Cerebral Palsy* (Ed.) Bax, M., Clayton-Jones, E. & Mac Keith, R. *Little Club Clinics in Developmental Medicine,* No. 2, pp. 133–136. London: Spastics Society.

Zangwill, O. L. (1960b) *Cerebral Dominance and Its Relation to Psychological Function.* Edinburgh: Oliver and Boyd.

Zausmer, E. & Tower, G. (1966) A quotient for the evaluation of motor development. *Physical Therapy,* **46,** 725–727.

Index